MADNESS
AND THE
BRAIN

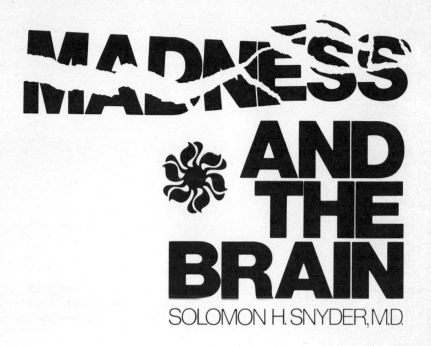

MADNESS AND THE BRAIN

SOLOMON H. SNYDER, M.D.

McGraw-Hill Book Company

New York • St. Louis • San Francisco • Düsseldorf • Mexico • Montreal
Panama • Paris • São Paulo • Tokyo • Toronto

First McGraw-Hill Paperback Edition, 1975.

2 3 4 5 6 7 8 9   MU MU   7 9 8 7 6 5

Library of Congress Cataloging in Publication Data

Snyder, Solomon H., date
   Madness and the brain

   Includes bibliographical references.
    1. Psychopharmacology. I. Title.
DNLM: 1. Psychopharmacology—Popular works.
QV77 S675d 1973
RC483.S57   615'.78   73-7763
ISBN 0-07-059521-6

To my teacher, Julius Axelrod

Contents

1

Why Madness?

This book is about drugs and the brain and the light they shed on the nature of "madness."

What is madness? I am concerned with the madness of those unfortunate individuals that we usually label as "insane" or "psychotic." We view such a person as so emotionally disturbed that he has lost contact with reality. We cannot reason with him. Nothing he says makes much sense. We have a feeling that his actions are going to be grossly unpredictable and that he might do things that could hurt himself or his loved ones. Our first inclination is to withdraw from him as a human being and focus upon how to have him committed to a mental hospital.

The average person feels uneasy when confronted with severe emotional disturbance, and he wishes he understood what was going on. Is madness a sentence for life? Are there different forms of psychosis, some in which the patient will recover in short order as contrasted to others in which the forecast is far more grave? What is going on in the sick one's brain? Why must he behave in these strange ways? Can any drugs alleviate the psychotic process in a more or less direct fashion? Are there a multiplicity of ways to be insane or are there only a few major mental illnesses?

Sadly, psychiatry has few answers to these questions. Before essaying any of them, we should first try to clarify the meaning of the words we use to refer to different forms of madness, insanity, or psychosis. In traditional psychiatric classifications there are only two major types of psychosis: schizophrenia and manic depressive psychosis.

Patients afflicted with manic depressive psychosis are either "high" or "low." Manic refers to the "high" times, when a patient is wildly exuberant, elated, talking a-mile-a-minute, filled with grandiose, though not bizarre, schemes for making money or benefiting mankind. He is constantly on the go, hardly sleeping or eating. He plays with words cleverly, constantly punning and making all sorts of clever associations. His mood of gaiety may even be infectious so that people see him as a delightful person until they become exhausted, disgusted, and ultimately worried by the incessant parade of words, ideas, and sheer physical movement.

What about depression? Everyone is depressed at one time or another. Some people are sufficiently depressed for long enough periods that they would benefit by psychiatric treatment. Depression becomes a form of psychosis only when it is severe enough to interrupt a person's activities at work and at home. An individual is said to be psychotically depressed when he is incapable of working and talks in a way suggesting that he seriously doubts whether he should go on living. When he cannot sleep at all and hardly eats, and when his forlorn and hopeless utterances are beginning to sound strange and inappropriate to what is going on in the world, then psychiatrists would tend to think that he may be depressed to a psychotic point.

Certain individuals experience episodes of mania at certain times and episodes of depression at other times; others may be depressed once or many times and never suffer from mania; and a limited number of patients have attacks of mania without ever being depressed. Whether mania and depression are distinct entities always, sometimes, or never is an unsettled question.

Though technically mania and depression are referred to in the usual psychiatric glossaries as psychotic disturbances, when most people think of insanity, madness, or psychosis they do not have in mind depression or elation. Instead they are thinking of individuals with a more bizarre and blatant loss of contact with reality, individuals whose thought processes are fragmented, convoluted, and awesome, people who hear voices and utter unworldly declarations and prophecies. In speaking of madness, the general public is referring to an illness which organized psychiatry has come to call "schizophrenia."

Why should anyone outside the mental health professions pay heed to schizophrenia, at least to the extent of reading a book about it? For one thing, the public has long been fascinated and frightened by schizophrenia. Few families are insulated from it. At least one percent of the population of every country on the earth suffers from the disease. These figures are obtained by very cautious estimates, usually derived by counting the number of people in mental hospitals.

Perhaps as many as ten times this number of people suffer from schizophrenia but escape hospitalization because the social network for detection, trapping, and incarceration of the deviant is inefficient, or simply because the nonhospitalized schizophrenics are not blatantly enough disturbed to warrant their separation from society.

Because the tendency to develop schizophrenia is probably genetically inherited, the number of individuals with a chance of "catching" schizophrenia is far greater than the number of overt schizophrenics. Thus some people have estimated that twenty to forty million Americans have at least some "taint" of schizophrenia, either in their genetic propensity to breed schizophrenics or perhaps to a limited extent in their own behavior. These statistics by themselves are enough reason for most of us to be concerned about schizophrenia and to learn as much about it as we can.

Schizophrenia is also fascinating because of the remarkable nature of the schizophrenic thought processes. The ways in which schizophrenics think and speak have attracted the attention of important writers and philosophers throughout the centuries. To describe it all too briefly, the essential disturbance in the schizophrenic is a disintegration of his sense of personal unity, the feeling that he is an individual, his experience of the self. In this crisis of identity, which makes the adolescent identity crisis seem trivial, the schizophrenic person is trying to come to grips with a threatened loss of his total being and in so doing is grappling with some of the most fundamental questions that man can ask. Who am I? Why do I exist? What is the meaning of my life? Of any life? What is the ultimate reality? Who is God? Am I God?

Thus schizophrenic individuals are the world's experts on the existential crises of humanity. They deal with such issues twenty-four hours a day. Their utterances are laden to overflowing with profound philosophic queries.

In recent years the question of "madness" has been thrust upon the public from the point of view of social morality. How should society treat its mentally ill? This sort of question has profound corollaries for our conception of the nature of mental illness. In the twentieth century there has been a growing concern for the rights of the mentally ill. Thomas Szasz, an eminent psychiatrist who has written extensively about these questions, has emphasized the extraordinary injustice of "committing" a person to an indefinite sentence in a mental institution. Often, criminals find themselves with the choice of pleading guilty to a crime or not guilty by reason of insanity. Depending on the nature of the crime, those who plead insanity sometimes find themselves locked up for indefinite and prolonged periods, much longer than they would have spent in jail.

Szasz has followed this line of reasoning to the ultimate conclusion: that the Western concept of mental illness is meaningless and refers to no concrete entity—mental illness is nothing but a "myth." According to Szasz, society labels as crazy anyone with deviant behavior in so arbitrary a fashion that the categories of mental illness become nothing but semantic artifices for maintaining the social order.

Phyllis Chesler has recently written a book called *Women and Madness,* developing a corollary of Szasz's thesis. She argues that women are labeled mentally ill insofar as they fail to accommodate themselves to the male chauvinist stereotype of the ideal female. Most men would like women to be passive, home-loving, and lacking in intellectual dynamism, in short, devoid of any threat to the dominant position of men in our society. Naturally, any woman who fails to conform to this stereotype is "deviant," and deviancy is readily equated with mental illness.

The Scottish psychiatrist Ronald Laing has gained widespread popularity by advancing a notion somewhat related to the thinking of Thomas Szasz. Laing argues that psychosis may not be altogether a myth, but neither is it something to be stamped out like pneumonia and cancer. Instead psychosis may well be a legitimate and productive means for dealing with the existential dilemmas that are imminent in modern life. Perhaps the conditions of life in the twentieth century are more "insane" than the mentally ill. Laing testifies to many instances in which the harrowing experience of a schizophrenic breakdown has been followed by the rebirth of a fruitful, enriched life style. He condemns the use of antischizophrenic tranquilizing drugs which, he maintains, abort the rejuvenating experience of the psychosis and instead confine the patient to a stifling existence altogether lacking in meaning.

A recent experimental study blatantly depicts the confused status of the diagnosis of madness. Dr. D. L. Rosenhan arranged to have eight people, all in normal mental health, admitted to a number of different mental hospitals throughout the country, including large state hospitals as well as small, private university hospitals. Though they mimicked a few symptoms of schizophrenia in order to secure admission, once admitted to the hospital they behaved in their usual fashion and did nothing at all to simulate mental illness.

Strikingly, the staff of every one of the mental hospitals treated these individuals as if they were schizophrenic and "explained" all their behavior in terms of their purported mental illness. Though they behaved normally while in the hospital, it was difficult for most of these individuals to secure release, and, when they were discharged, it was not with a clean bill of health, but with the diagnosis "schizophrenia, in remission."

The writings of Szasz and Laing, and too many Kafkaesque encounters with the mental health profession reminiscent of Dr. Rosenhan's study, have bewildered the general public. What do you do if a friend behaves bizarrely? Will turning him over to the psychiatrist help him or harm him? Will psychiatric treatment restore him to normal function or destroy his potential for real happiness? Is there really such thing as psychosis? What does it mean when someone is diagnosed as being schizophrenic? Is he merely being railroaded into a hospital as a victim of some politically oppressive scheme, much as the Russian government has used psychiatric confinement as a means of silencing political dissent?

Laing and Szasz and others have raised important questions about the way society views and deals with madness. However cogent their arguments, they still do not negate the fact of mental illness, the existence of psychotic disturbance in many millions of America, and the concrete reality of entities such as schizophrenia and manic depressive psychosis. As will become amply evident throughout this book, there is abundant genetic and clinical evidence that the disease entity of schizophrenia, as well as other psychotic disturbances, is genuine. The difficulty of the psychiatric community stems from the lack of a simple physical indicator of the disease. There is no germ which can be cultured or examined under the microscope. There is no chemical test in blood or urine that will provide a definitive answer. One is left with the task of judging the patient's feelings and thoughts as evidenced in his speech and actions.

It is important to recognize and to know basic information about psychosis for several reasons. First, as already mentioned, no human being is remote from the plight of the psychotically disturbed. There are also more positive reasons for wanting to know all there is to be known about mental illness. Perhaps one of the most exciting aspects is the progress that modern science is now making toward understanding the nature of severe mental illness. There now exist valuable drugs which alleviate the symptoms of schizophrenia. Other drugs are known which can provoke symptoms closely mimicking those of schizophrenia. By knowing how the antischizophrenic drugs act in the brain to alleviate psychotic symptoms and by knowing how other drugs produce mental disturbances akin to schizophrenia, we may be coming close to an understanding of what is askew in the brains of schizophrenics. Not only is schizophrenia a real disease or group of diseases, but it may be possible in the not-too-distant future to understand its fundamental base just as clearly as we can identify the causative organism in bacterial pneumonia.

Knowing all about bacterial pneumonia is important for the physician but not particularly critical for the layman. Schizophrenia, by contrast, is a major concern of all mankind. Sigmund Freud repeatedly demonstrated that, by comprehending the psychology of the emotionally disturbed, one could draw major inferences about the thinking and feeling processes of all human beings. Although Freud's conceptions were all at a psychological level, he was convinced that a biological basis existed for the major mental disturbances, especially schizophrenia. Freud's fondest dream was to see the psychological facts about mental functioning in illness and in health linked to the chemical and physical architecture of the brain.

During the past few decades knowledge of the biology of the brain has accumulated at a rapidly escalating pace. Basic facts about brain functioning can now be linked to mental disease by studying the mechanism of action of drugs which change normal or abnormal reality in remarkable ways. It now seems possible to begin an integration of this biological information with the psychology of the well and unwell mind. There are no final answers today, but there are strong hints which tempt one toward provocative speculation and hope. And that is what this book is all about.

2

Antischizophrenic Drugs

Yes, Virginia, there are antischizophrenic drugs. Of course, these drugs don't fully cure schizophrenics, but they certainly do something to the disease process in a very specific and selective way. They are not merely sedatives to ease the patient of restless, hyperanxious activity or, more to the point, to ease his custodian by essentially bludgeoning the patient into semiconsciousness.

Oh, surely everybody knows that psychiatrists, like all other doctors, have their bag full of tricks. There are stimulants to perk you up if you are feeling downtrodden; there are tranquilizers to ease your anxiety about asking the boss for a raise; and there are a seemingly endless assortment of pills to get you peacefully and obliviously through the night. But knowing that John or Mary, who has had a "nervous breakdown," are being treated by a psychiatrist with "tranquilizers" which seem to keep them functioning is not at all the same as appreciating that their disease (schizophrenia) has been altered in some essential fashion by drugs which do more than bring about quiet, calm, "good" behavior. Such drugs should surely qualify, more than all other known therapeutic agents, as "miracle drugs." They are called the phenothiazine tranquilizers.

A Story of Serendipity

My dictionary says that serendipity is "the faculty of making desirable but unsought-for discoveries by accident." In science there is a long tradition which emphasizes that serendipitous discoveries are the hallmark of brilliant scientists. Most scientific discoveries are unexpected and rarely predicted. The astute investigator is intrigued by an experimental result which looks rather peculiar. He can see situations in which a seemingly unimportant piece of data, looking more like the outcome of poorly washed glassware than of the operations of some fundamental law of nature, can, in fact, point toward some conceptual advance. Most great scientists feel that processes like these underlie all their important breakthroughs. Louis Pasteur epitomized this attitude and emphasized that "chance favors the prepared mind." Others have wondered whether serendipity originates more in the romanticized reminiscences of aging eminent scientists than in the process of research itself and have defined serendipity as a "'portmanteau' word signifying a mental state [combining] serenity and stupidity . . . or the sort of thing that happens to you when on a dull day collecting fossils you find instead a beautiful woman who proves to be neither geologist nor archeologist."

Whether serendipity is something which touches the

divine or is simply silly, there is little doubt that something akin to it played a major role in the advent of the phenothiazine drugs into psychiatry as important therapy for schizophrenia.

Phenothiazine itself, the basic nucleus of the phenothiazine antischizophrenic drugs, was first synthesized by a German chemist in 1880. It was used for years, and is still used to a limited extent, for the therapy of worm infections, especially those which invade the gastrointestinal tract. There was little interest in developing new uses for and derivatives of phenothiazine until the early 1940s. At that time one of the major breakthroughs in drug development took place—the appearance of antihistamines, a discovery for which the Italian pharmacologist Daniel Bovet was to receive a Nobel Prize. Drug companies were agog. Not only were there potential customers among the many millions of hay fever sufferers, but, as with any new phenomenon in medicine, physicians and scientists became curious about the multiple aspects of normal and disturbed body function in which histamine might play a role and in which antihistamine drugs might accordingly be valuable therapeutic agents. Histamine is a chemical stored in many cells throughout the body and released in allergic reactions, causing many of the symptoms of human allergy. Antihistamines block the effects of histamine. Antihistamines have been used in treating conditions ranging from asthma, high blood pressure, low blood pressure, and shock to the common cold. Indeed, for many years, treating the common cold with antihistamines, a means now known to be quite ineffective, has accounted for the great bulk of their manufacture and sale. Not surprisingly, the basic phenothiazine structure was among many chemical structures which were incorporated into the fairly simple "chemical formula" which labeled a compound as having the characteristics of an antihistamine. The first major antihistaminic phenothiazine, promethazine, was introduced in 1945. Its trade name in the United States is Phenergan.

In the 1940s surgeons too were eager to exploit the antihistamines one way or another. The French surgeon Henri Laborit had been studying mechanisms which might underlie surgical shock for some years. The problem is a straightforward one. Many patients given enough of a general anesthetic to render them sufficiently unconscious and immobile for surgery fall into a state of shock, which often proves fatal. The major symptom in shock is a marked decrease in blood pressure. It is well known that injected histamine can evoke a lowering of blood pressure. Laborit reasoned that histamine release, perhaps in response to the stress of the surgical procedure, might be responsible for the shock and therefore that antihistamines might alleviate it. The antihistamine promethazine didn't do much to the blood pressure of his patients, but Laborit noticed something that seemed more interesting. He observed that, when given several hours before the operation, promethazine rendered his patients sleepy and less apprehensive than normal, though not at all confused. It seemed like the sort of drug which might make anesthesia more effective in lower doses; hence, with less likelihood of shock resulting.

Morphine had been used in the past for such a purpose. But morphine, unlike the antihistamines, depresses the breathing centers and, when combined with the trauma of surgery in a sick patient, might join with the lowered blood pressure to precipitate sudden death. Besides, morphine often confuses patients and makes them nauseous. Thus Laborit was quite enthusiastic about the value of promethazine as a preoperative medication "for reasons we had not expected. Our patients are calm, somewhat somnolent, relaxed and look rested . . . even after major operations they are never excited, not complaining, and appear to really suffer less."

Promethazine continues to this day to be used as a preoperative medication and also serves as a convenient and relatively safe sleeping pill for children. The commercial potential of Laborit's new way of using antihistamines did not go unnoticed for long. Physicians and patients have been well aware of the sedative properties of antihistamines ever since their introduction into clinical medicine. In fact, even now sedation is looked on as the most troublesome side effect of antihistamines. Many allergic patients prefer to suffer with the worst of their hay fever rather than walk about all day in a drowsy state. Most drug companies utilized several animal tests to detect any sedative properties in potential antihistaminic drugs, properties such as their ability to prolong sleep induced by barbiturates or to impair some kinds of motor performance in rats, such as climbing a rope. Compounds which were found to be mainly sedating agents were summarily discarded.

Within a year of Laborit's publishing his work with promethazine in surgical anesthesia, the French drug company Specia revamped their screening program for antihistamines. They reexamined the great numbers of compounds synthesized during the preceding years which had been banished to basement storerooms because they were basically sedatives and had only weak antihistaminic effects. Now their screening tests became directed toward compounds which would sedate an animal and thereby impair his performance of some task, yet not put him to sleep too readily. Besides screening old compounds, the Specia chemist Paul Charpentier, an expert in the synthesis of phenothiazines, prepared a number of new phenothiazine derivatives. One of these appeared especially promising in animals and was quickly dispatched to Laborit for testing in humans. Charpentier called it chlorpromazine, because it came from an already known phenothiazine, promazine, and was formed by the simple addition of a chlorine atom.

Laborit was extraordinarily impressed with chlorpromazine. It did exactly what he wanted. His patients were rendered calm and tranquil but were still alert, and there were no serious side effects. Chlorpromazine was the first of what would prove to be the antischizophrenic agents and the one still most widely used in clinical psychiatry, so that Laborit's comments are of special interest: "In doses of 50–100 mg intravenously, it provokes not any loss in consciousness, not any change in the patient's mentality but a slight tendency to sleep and above all 'disinterest' for all that goes on around him."

Laborit was dead right about chlorpromazine as an adjunct to surgical anesthesia. It remains a drug of choice for this purpose today. More important, Laborit was astute enough to recognize that such an agent, a drug which can turn off the world and its onslaught of sensory stimulation without confusing the patient or putting him to sleep, might have uses in numerous fields besides surgery.

In the first clinical publication on chlorpromazine he suggested, "These facts let us foresee certain indications for this drug in psychiatry." A dynamic man, Laborit quickly got the drug into the hands of several psychiatrists in Paris. One of his colleagues gave it to a manic patient with only limited success. Psychiatrists at another hospital administered the drug in very small doses and were unimpressed. However, within a few months Jean Delay and Pierre Deniker treated numerous patients with a variety of diagnoses with adequate doses. They tried the drug with hyperactive manic patients, with retarded depressives, with anxious neurotics, and with all sorts of schizophrenics. Some patients responded dramatically, and it was clear that what they had in common was the disease schizophrenia.

The race was on. Within a few years chlorpromazine was being administered to schizophrenic patients throughout the United States. The atmosphere of mental hospitals everywhere was affected radically. The number of patients who remained in hospitals for long periods with wildly agitated behavior, smearing feces and so forth, decreased strikingly, sometimes to the vanishing point. Instead of looking forward to a stay of years in a state mental hospital, the average schizophrenic in the United States could now hope to be discharged, well enough to function in society, in about two months. Accordingly, after the introduction of chlorpromazine, the number of patients in state mental hospitals began falling so rapidly that people made predictions that soon it might be possible to close down all such institutions.

Slow to Catch On

In contrast to the phenothiazines, which were first administered to humans in a small hospital in Paris in the spring of 1952, and which in two years had become the drugs of choice in the treatment of schizophrenia all over the civilized world, *Rauwolfia*, the other major type of antischizophrenic drug, had to mark time, not years, but centuries, before it was recognized by organized psychiatry.

Rauwolfia is simply an extract of the Indian snakeroot plant, whose botanical name is *Rauwolfia serpentina*. It has been used in India for almost two thousand years in treating numerous conditions, ranging from snakebite (hence the name *"serpentina"*), to various diseases of the circulation (most of which probably represented high blood pressure), up to insanity. Its value in the treatment of psychosis was so well accepted in Indian folk medicine that one of the Indian names for extracts of the plant is *pagla-ka-dawa*, which means "insanity herb."

In 1931 two Indian physicians, Ganneth Sen and Katrick Bose, reported the systematic study of *Rauwolfia* as a treatment for high blood pressure and for psychoses. Over the next twenty years there were sporadic reports of the value of *Rauwolfia* in lowering blood pressure and in treating insanity, but few people paid attention and the drug remained unknown to Western medicine. The breakthrough that brought *Rauwolfia* into sidespread attention came when chemists at the Ciba Drug Company in Switzerland isolated the chemical from the *Rauwolfia* plant which was responsible for its ability to lower blood pressure. They called the drug reserpine.

Isolating and synthesizing a pure chemical from a plant gives one a "new drug," something which can be patented and marketed at a high profit. Ciba was eager to promote this new drug as an antihypertensive agent; but they didn't seem to be particularly interested in its use for psychiatric patients. The initiative came, not from the drug company, but from Dr. Nathan Kline, an irrepressible, enthusiastic American psychiatrist, and one of the founders of psychopharmacology in this country. He had read of the Indian traditions and persuaded the Ciba Company to finance an evaluation of reserpine in psychiatry. Kline is a fast worker. Within a year he had treated seven hundred patients with reserpine and was confident that here was an important drug in the therapy for schizophrenia. He presented his findings early in 1954 at about the same time that chlorpromazine was being introduced into the United States. Like chlorpromazine, reserpine seemed to bring about miracles in mental hospitals throughout the country. One of the better reports in 1954 on the effects of the reserpine depicts the glad tidings:

> Since the advent of therapy with reserpine . . . patients have undergone a metamorphosis from raging, combating, unsociable persons to cooperative, friendly, cheerful, sociable, relatively quiet persons who are admittable to psychotherapy and rehabilitative measures. Hyperactive patients have become quiet, sedate, and cooperative in their behavior. Noisy patients have become quiet, while withdrawn and depressed patients have become alert and cheerful in their demeanor.

The comment that the drug both calms hyperactive patients and activates the withdrawn ones is quite important. It emphasizes that the drug is not by any means a mere sedative, but must be doing something that is specifically antischizophrenic. The drug drastically altered all custodial procedures in the hospitals and exhilarated the physicians. "On the wards where the patients are receiving reserpine, seclusion, restraint of all types, sedative and electroconvulsive therapy have been almost eliminated. It seems incredible that a drug can replace electroconvulsive therapy in this manner, but apparently such a drug has been found, and we expect it to revolutionize and facilitate modern psychiatric treatment.''

Chemically, the phenothiazines and reserpine are very different drugs. Moreover, their actions in the brain are somewhat different, although they accomplish the same effects within particular, critical groups of nerves in the brain. Though they are both effective antischizophrenic agents, reserpine tends to have more side effects, particularly lowering of blood pressure; so that, in modern psychiatric practice, phenothiazines and their relatives are far and away the most widely prescribed drugs for schizophrenia. Their effect in the treatment of mental illness and their influence upon society has been enormous.

Impact of Antischizophrenic Drugs

In 1955 about 560,000 patients populated the mental hospitals of America. One out of every two hospital beds in the United States was occupied by a psychiatric patient, an unpleasant bit of information known to too few people. Fully half of those patients were schizophrenic, the remainder being spread among an assortment of diagnoses, including alcoholism, cerebral arteriosclerosis, and simply old people who had no one else to take care of them. At the rate at which the population of the mental hospitals was increasing, it was estimated that by 1971 the total number would be about 750,000 patients. But something remarkable happened. In 1954–1955 when the antischizophrenic drugs, the phenothiazines and reserpine, were introduced into state mental hospitals in America, the old trend began to change rapidly.

The optimistic feelings of the staffs of mental hospitals about the new drugs have been well born out by the statistics. In 1971, 330,000 psychiatric patients inhabited the state mental hospitals—less than half the projected hospital population of 750,000. What makes this even more dramatic is the fact that between 1955 and 1971, while the sharp fall in the number of patients residing in the hospitals was taking place, the number of admissions to the hospitals was doubling. This was not due to any epidemic of mental illness during this period, but because people have become more astute in recognizing the symptoms of mental illness, and have at the same time become far more optimistic about the prospects for something positive happening in the hospital. Perhaps the most positive thing which has taken place is that the average duration of hospitalization has fallen so precipitously that schizophrenic patients can expect to remain in the hospital for only about two months.

Let us translate the numbers into human considerations. Since the introduction of these drugs, the "snake-pit" atmosphere of the back wards of mental hospitals, with walls and floors covered with human excrement, and filled twenty-four hours a day with terror-laden shrieking, essentially exist no more. Perhaps just as important as the state of mind of the patients themselves is the salutory effect of antischizophrenic drugs upon the attitudes and feelings of the families of the mentally ill. And there are many such families. At least one percent of the United States population is overtly schizophrenic by anyone's criteria; while about four times as many individuals suffer from schizophrenia but have gone undiagnosed for one reason or another. For these families, prior to the phenothiazine revolution, the full realization of the nature of the illness of their loved one brought with it a feeling akin to a death sentence. Chances were all too good that the patient, once packed up and sent off to a state hospital, would never return. Now there is no need for such pessimism. The great majority of schizophrenics, after hospitalization, return to society to lead functional lives. Some have residual symptoms and are never fully "normal," and some may have to be rehospitalized again and again. But a good number improve to such a point that, for all practical purposes, they can be thought of as cured.

Are You Convinced?

By constantly harping on the fact that phenothiazine drugs and reserpine influence the disease process itself, I have been asking the reader to take a rather hefty assertion on faith. Many psychiatrists remained unconvinced of the antischizophrenic action of these drugs for years and years, and with good reason. While these agents were introduced in 1952, the evidence for their antischizophrenic action was not really solid until about 1964. Why such a long delay? Surely there must have been many psychiatrists studying the drugs and publishing their findings? Indeed, in the two decades since chlorpromazine was first administered to psychiatric patients, there have been upwards of ten thousand publications. Sadly, most of these are what scientists refer to as "uncontrolled" studies. In an uncontrolled drug trial, the physician administers the drug to a number of his patients and then reports the extent to which they benefit from the medication. At first blush, this might seem fairly reasonable. However, a moment's reflection reveals grave weaknesses.

The most prominent of these weaknesses is the so-called "placebo effect." Countless studies have proved that patients with almost any sort of medical or psychiatric disease will feel much improved if the doctor gives them a pill or capsule containing no active drug at all, usually just some sugar, and tells them that the medication will make them better. This type of pill is called a placebo. Placebos work just as well for such obviously "real" symptoms as the pain of cancer or the aching of a slipped disc, as for more "psychosomatic" complaints such as headaches or simple anxiety. Some shrewd investigators have even demonstrated that patients with neurotic symptoms are markedly improved when treated with placebos, even though the physician tells the patient that he is receiving a sugar pill which contains no active medication. In these cases, the patients who have received the placebo do significantly better than individuals who are given verbal reassurance as emotional support. Oh, the power of a pill!

Because patients with psychiatric symptoms are so suggestible and profoundly influenced by anything the doctor tells them to put into their mouths, it is easy to see why uncontrolled studies of drugs in psychiatry should be viewed with considerable skepticism. In reviewing hundreds of studies of psychiatric drugs, researchers have found that uncontrolled studies invariably report more positive effects from drugs tested than controlled studies. In controlled studies, the influence of the drug on the psychiatric symptoms is compared to whatever change in symptoms occurs when the same or comparable patients receive a placebo. Indeed, there are many instances in which uncontrolled studies have provided enthusiastic reports about drugs which were subsequently shown to be altogether useless.

Clearly, in evaluating the thousands of investigations of phenothiazines or reserpine in schizophrenic patients, we must be wary of studies in which placebo groups were not employed. Actually, giving a sugar pill placebo is not an altogether sure way of barring against error. Most drugs elicit a number of effects other than the desired therapeutic ones. These side effects are easily detected by the physician. Accordingly, a so-called controlled study in which some patients are receiving a sugar pill and others the active drug will no longer be controlled as soon as the physician, consciously or unconsciously, detects the side effects of the experimental drug. For soon he will unknowingly be more energetic and optimistic in dealing with the patients who are receiving the "real" drug and whom the doctor therefore expects to improve the most. Because patients are so readily influenced by suggestion, the subtlest differences in the physician's attitude may be enough to produce different responses in the two groups of patients, even where the "active drug" is really no better than the placebo.

To make sure that the conscious or unconscious feelings of the doctor will not determine the response to the drug, the best experimenters always include "active placebos." An active placebo is a drug which will reproduce the side effects of the drug being studied, but which presumably displays none of its therapeutic actions. For instance, if one wished to evaluate the effectiveness of Alka-Seltzer as an antacid, the ideal placebo would be a pill which fizzes gloriously but which has no antacid effects of its own. In studies of antischizophrenic drugs—especially chlorpromazine, which has a pronounced sedating action—the active placebo generally used is a barbiturate, such as phenobarbital, which is similarly sedating.

All these considerations are terribly important, because, without careful controls for placebo effects and other factors, it is impossible to tease apart the variegated changes in the behavior of psychiatric patients when they are treated with psychoactive drugs. How does one decide what is the primary effect of the drug and what is only secondary? With the antischizophrenic drugs, there has been continual debate ever since their introduction as to whether or not they interacted directly with the schizophrenic processes in the brains of the mentally ill, or whether they did something to the brain unrelated to schizophrenia but which, in turn, helped the schizophrenic to accommodate to his environment. Authorities of comparable eminence have espoused each side of the controversy.

Antischizophrenic or Antianxiety?

Many skeptics argue that phenothiazines are simply supersedatives, easing the overwhelming anxiety of schizophrenics. If so, barbiturates would be just as good for schizophrenics. However, in many carefully performed studies comparing phenobarbital and phenothiazines, the phenothiazines always have triumphed. Indeed the barbiturates invariably fail to produce any more improvement in schizophrenic patients than a sugar pill or no drug treatment at all. By contrast, reserpine and all the major phenothiazine drugs are clearly effective in improving the overall mental health of schizophrenics.

The fact that the phenothiazines are more effective than phenobarbital suggests that they are not acting simply by sedating the patients or relieving their anxiety. Of course, someone might argue that phenobarbital is not the ideal drug for easing anxiety. In the case of overwhelming anxiety bordering on and sometimes exceeding panic in schizophrenic patients, perhaps phenobarbital is simply too weak and the phenothiazines are more powerful. Indeed, in studies of neurotic outpatients, it is difficult to demonstrate any marked beneficial effects of phenobarbital. The more widely prescribed antianxiety tranquilizers, such as chlordiazepoxide (Librium) and diazepam (Valium), do a much better job than phenobarbital. If the key to relieving schizophrenic symptoms is control of panic and anxiety, one would expect drugs like Librium and Valium to be effective. However, several psychiatrists have evaluated these agents and found them to be no more effective than placebos in easing the plight of the schizophrenic patient.

The anxiety question can be attacked from yet another point of view. If the phenothiazines are acting to relieve anxiety, one would expect them to be useful in treating anxiety neurosis and perhaps other neuroses. Many physicians prescribe phenothiazines to their neurotic patients for this purpose. Unfortunately, while phenothiazines may be the wonder drugs of the century for schizophrenia, several studies have shown that they are quite poor if not altogether ineffective in treating neuroses with varying degrees of manifest anxiety. Because the phenothiazines cause many more side effects than the antianxiety drugs and because the adverse effects of the phenothiazines are considerably more dangerous, authorities now feel that it is quite unwise to treat neurotics with the phenothiazine drugs. They have their place. That place is schizophrenia.

Psychiatrists enamored of the notion that phenothiazines act by calming down patients have decided that hyperactive patients should be treated with sedating type of phenothiazines, while withdrawn patients should receive nonsedating "activating" phenothiazines. Careful evaluation of many patients has essentially disproven this simple-minded saw. When treated with a sedating phenothiazine such as chlorpromazine, not only do hyperactive patients become quieter, but withdrawn patients become more active. The same thing happens with the so-called activating phenothiazines.

Which Symptoms Succumb?

Yet another way to measure the unique influence of the phenothiazines upon schizophrenic symptoms is to dissect the individual symptoms of the disease and assess how each responds to the drug. This complex task has been undertaken by several groups of investigators, usually employing many hundreds of patients located in several hospitals in the United States. In this way, results are more likely to be representative of schizophrenic patients in general, rather than an accidental grouping of peculiarities at any particular hospital.

A simple way of summing up the different responses

of schizophrenic symptoms to these drugs is to look at them in terms of Bleuler's classification of fundamental, accessory, and nonschizophrenic symptoms. Table 1 summarizes the results of a large number of studies, many of which describe the various symptoms in different ways. However, in Table 1, which is derived from Dr. John Davis's elegant and careful analysis, they have all been translated into a standard description. There is little doubt that the schizophrenic symptoms improve more with drug treatment than do nonschizophrenic symptoms. Among the nonschizophrenic symptoms are some which have been advanced by many psychiatrists as ways in which phenothiazines could indirectly improve the behavior of schizophrenics. We have already discussed how relief of anxiety–tension–agitation might secondarily ease the pain of the basis schizophrenic symptoms. Similarly, one might expect all schizophrenics to be depressed about their lot in life. Sandor Rado even suggested that the inability to experience any pleasure is at the basis of schizophrenia. However, any depressive feelings which schizophrenics might bear do not seem to improve with drug treatment.

In striking contrast, both the fundamental and accessory symptoms of schizophrenia do improve under the influence of the drugs. In summarizing results of a large number of patients, it appears that there is somewhat greater improvement in the fundamental than in the accessory symptoms, although this distinction is not ironclad. One would not expect it to be easy to differentiate improvement in fundamental and accessory symptoms. If one agrees that the accessory symptoms, the hallucinations, delusions, and so on, derive from the more fundamental disorders of thinking and feeling,

TABLE 1

ANALYSIS OF SYMPTOM SENSITIVITY TO PHENOTHIAZINES

Bleuler's Classification of Schizophrenic Symptoms	Response to Treatment
FUNDAMENTAL	
Thought disorder	+++
Blunted affect–indifference	++
Withdrawal–retardation	++
Autistic behavior–mannerisms	++
ACCESSORY	
Hallucinations	++
Paranoid ideation	+
Grandiosity	+
Hostility–belligerence	+
Resistiveness–uncooperativeness	+
NONSCHIZOPHRENIC	
Anxiety–tension–agitation	0
Guilt–depression	0
Disorientation	0
Somatization	0

one would expect the fundamental symptoms to be affected first, after which the accessory symptoms would tend to evaporate of themselves. This would explain neatly a slightly greater improvement in fundamental than in accessory symptoms.

Some scientists have directly examined, by psychological tests, the influence of phenothiazines on fundamental symptoms in schizophrenic patients. For instance, schizophrenics tend to be "overinclusive" in their thinking processes (combining unrelated ideas in sentences, for example). Phenothiazines definitely reduce this disturbance of thinking. Another aspect of the schizophrenic disorder is the tendency to think concretely rather than abstractly. Again, phenothiazines enhance the ability of schizophrenics to handle abstractions.

The Practicalities

Everyone agrees on a number of concrete facts regarding the effects of antischizophrenic drugs on schizophrenic patients. These are worth revealing in some detail, because a number of them have cogent bearing upon the issue of how these agents do their job.

One striking fact which has rendered the drug therapy of schizophrenic patients an elusive art is the enormous variability in dosage of phenothiazines required in individual patients. This variability has been best documented with chlorpromazine, the mother drug. Many patients do quite well on 75 milligrams of chlorpromazine, while others often require as much as 2000 milligrams. How is the poor psychiatrist to determine the requirements of his patient? His only possible approach, which is currently the standard therapeutic regimen, is to increase the amount of the drug until maximal therapeutic benefit occurs—a point beyond which further increases in the medication fail to be of benefit. This is without question a tricky business. It is hard enough to monitor patient improvement at all. Deciding that the rate of improvement is slowing down, that the patient is leveling off and so on, is not easy. Doctors do their best, and no one is ever sure about the optimum amount of drug for his patient. Everyone does agree that this optimum varies enormously among patients.

What might account for the difference in dosage requirements? The simplest explanation would be that patients vary greatly in the rate at which their bodies destroy the drugs, a phenomenon which is well known with many medications. Thus one might argue that with the same amount of a phenothiazine in the brain all patients would manifest the same therapeutic response. However, any two patients might differ tenfold in the amount of drug which must be taken in order to attain that ideal brain level. It should be simple enough to answer this question. All one need do is measure blood levels of the drug. Unfortunately, blood levels of the phenothiazine tranquilizers have turned out to be quite low and not accessible to easy measurement.

Main Effects, Side Effects

One way or another, most, if not all, schizophrenics improve with reserpine and the phenothiazine tranquilizers. The rate of improvement is similar with all the drugs of these classes. Patients' overall behavior becomes less disordered gradually over a period of about four to six weeks, after which the beneficial effects tend to plateau. A practical lesson to be drawn from this item of information is that physicians should not hastily conclude that a given drug was not effective after only a brief one-week trial.

For many patients improvement is so dramatic that one might claim that they are "cured." If one is cautious and maintains that schizophrenia is a genetic illness which can never really be fully cured, he could describe the total absence of symptoms by saying that the patient has experienced an impressive "remission." Other patients are never fully symptom free, but are so much better that they can leave the hospital and function admirably in society. An unfortunate minority appears less deranged with the drugs but is never well enough to leave the hospital.

With all patients, but most especially with those who have had a total remission, the question arises of how long they should continue to take the medication. Is this like insulin and the diabetic? Is a schizophrenic sentenced to his phenothiazine tranquilizer for life? No one knows the answer for certain. However, all psychiatrists agree that the patient in glorious remission would be wise to avoid the tendency to cast off his phenothiazine crutches. Numerous studies have examined just what happens when medication is terminated and a placebo is substituted in patients who seem to be all better. The frequency of relapses in such individuals is far greater than in comparable groups in which the drug treatment was continued. Because of findings such as these, some psychiatrists feel that a patient with schizophrenia is sentenced to a lifetime of his medicines. I am not sure. Some patients may require the drugs for the rest of their lives while others may not. It is possible that, after a patient has been symptom free for some time, the medication may be gradually tapered down and ultimately discontinued. For some patients the schizophrenic derangement may turn off following the brief psychotic episode after which normal mental functioning is permanently restored. For others the disturbance will always be present and is only toned down by the drugs. With yet another class of individuals, the diseased alterations may revert after treatment to full normality—which however is tenuous, so that in the absence of maintenance with phenothiazines they may flip back to a schizophrenic state. An especially intriguing possibility is that certain schizophrenics might be better off without drugs than with them.

Different Drugs, Different Nuances

Reserpine was the single active ingredient isolated from the *Rauwolfia* plant. A few analogues of reserpine were synthesized by drug companies, but none have gained wide favor in psychiatry. Because of its potent blood pressure–lowering actions, reserpine itself is hardly used any longer. By contrast, the phenothiazines have proliferated seemingly without end. Many thousands have been prepared and a fairly large number are commonly employed in psychiatry. In terms of their ability to improve the overall behavior of schizophrenics, most of the phenothiazines are similarly effective. Differences lie largely in the realm of side effects.

As already discussed, chlorpromazine is quite sedating. Normal people who ingest substantial doses report that they feel like they are walking around in a fog, somewhat drowsy, not confused, but not optimally responsive to what is going on about them. About half of the phenothiazine tranquilizers marketed in the United States have sedative properties similar to those of chlorpromazine. The other half are nonsedating and, in fact, have been described by their manufacturers as "activating." It is possible that they have some moderate stimulant, alerting effects, although these are by no means profound. These non-sedating phenothiazines appear to be equally effective as the sedating agents in treating all forms of schizophrenia. Here then is a point in support of those who argue that the antischizophrenic effects of phenothiazines have nothing to do with their sedating properties. The drowsiness produced by the sedating phenothiazines does tend to ease with time. However, the drugs continue to relieve the schizophrenic symptoms with no abatement in efficacy.

The sedating phenothiazines also tend to lower blood pressure, especially when patients stand up. When first treated with the drugs, many individuals will faint almost every time they arise from bed. Tolerance develops also to this particular side effect. Liver and blood abnormalities rarely occur with phenothiazine treatment. The sedating phenothiazines require considerably higher doses than the activating ones. In fact, there seems to be some rough parallel between the size of the dose required and the degree of sedation.

The least sedation occurs with some very new agents, the butyrophenones (see appendix), whose chemical structure is different from that of the phenothiazines, but whose pharmacologic effects are essentially the same. The butyrophenones are the most potent of the antischizophrenic drugs. One can treat patients with a butyrophenone at only one-hundredth the dose that would be required if chlorpromazine were used.

Like Parkinsonism

The most frequent types of side effects, which are at the same time the most intriguing and of considerable theoretical significance, are those which resemble the symptoms of Parkinson's disease, that condition occurring usually in middle-aged individuals in which there is a progressive inability to move any of the body's voluntary muscles. One of the most characteristic features of Parkinson's disease is a rhythmic tremor. The tremor occurs at rest and subsides when the patient actively and voluntarily moves his limbs. Although unattractive, a tremor is something most people can live with.

A more serious disability is the general stiffness of all the muscles and great difficulty in moving. Typically, this is expressed as a staring and motionless facial expression, a monotonous voice, a general slowness of all movements, and a curious lack of the little spontaneous changes in posture that are so characteristic of the normal individual. When this stiffening of the muscles comes on gradually, it is readily mistaken for a mild depression which is so common in middle-aged people. They have the freezing of the facial muscles as well as a glum and taciturn attitude. But as these changes progress inexorably, patients may become totally immobile wheelchair cases. They often die of infections such as pneumonia which develop largely as a result of their immobility.

Since its description by James Parkinson in 1817, this disease has been a grave frustration to physicians. Despite all their ministrations, the symptoms become worse and worse with time. Many of the 500,000 to 1,000,000 Americans with Parkinson's disease could anticipate the fatal sentence of life frozen in a bed or wheelchair, like Lot's wife in Sodom. Since 1967, treatment with L-dopa, one of the true miracle drugs of the twentieth century, has sprung thousands of patients with this disease out of their wheelchairs. The theoretical implications of L-dopa, its mechanism of action in Parkinson's disease, and its relevance to psychiatric illness will be touched on in later chapters.

With reserpine and the phenothiazine tranquilizers, Parkinson-like symptoms occur quite frequently, sometimes in as much as eighty-five percent of patients. Some of these patients will have symptoms indistinguishable from those of non–drug induced Parkinson's disease. However, there are several other symptoms, related to Parkinson's disease and presumably mediated by the same parts of the brain, which occur uniquely with the drugs. One symptom which is particularly exasperating to psychiatrists is akathisia. Patients appear restless and describe a peculiar "itchiness" in their muscles. They can't sit still and will pace endlessly up and down the halls of the hospital. Too frequently, the psychiatrist surmises that the patient is becoming agitated and needs more drug to quiet him down. Of course, since we are dealing with a drug side effect, the akathisia then worsens and soon a vicious cycle is under way.

Another related side effect consists of uncoordinated spasmodic movements of the body and the limbs. Occasionally the patient's back will become rigidly and most uncomfortably arched backwards. The neck may screw up to the side and the patient's eyes roll up in their sockets. Here too arise mistakes on the physician's part. These symptoms are frequently misdiagnosed as catatonic stuporous manifestations. If the patient is in a remission of his schizophrenic symptoms, the psychiatrist may think he is witnessing hysterical seizures, dramatic, semivoluntary efforts of the patient to gain the physician's attention, to keep him in the hospital and out of the clutches of an unappetizing family situation at home.

Because the Parkinsonian-like side effects of phenothiazines are so disconcerting and so frequent, drug manufacturers have synthesized tens of thousands and maybe even hundreds of thousands of analogues in an effort to obtain drugs which would be effective in treating schizophrenia without producing these side effects. Such searches for side effect–free drugs are a standard practice in the pharmaceutical industry and are often eminently successful. Strangely enough, with the phenothiazine tranquilizers it does not seem possible to develop an agent free of the Parkinsonian side effects. In fact there appears to be an intimate parallelism between the potency of the drugs in treating the symptoms of schizophrenia and their ability to produce these side effects.

By its very nature, schizophrenia is a uniquely human illness. There are no animal models of the disease, a fact which has stymied researchers for centuries. Things are quite different with Parkinson's disease. It is a straightforward neurological condition which can be readily simulated in several animal species. The biochemical changes in the brain which give rise to Parkinsonian symptoms are becoming increasingly apparent to researchers. The nature of the link between inducing the symptoms of Parkinsonism and reducing those of schizophrenia is becoming tantalizingly close to the grasp of brain scientists.

Keeping the World at Bay

The great body of evidence thus strongly suggests that reserpine and the phenothiazines are doing something very special in schizophrenic patients. Since they affect schizophrenic symptoms in a selective way, the simplest conclusion to draw is that they are acting in the brain at the sites of *the* schizophrenic dysfunction. Accordingly, if one knew at which place or chemical reaction the drugs exerted their effect, one would have localized the defect in schizophrenia. We must be cautious before jumping to such a conclusion. Even though phenothiazines might have a true anti-schizophrenic action, it need not be exerted directly at the brain locus of schizophrenia. The drugs might well act on some other area which in turn influences the schizophrenic mechanisms.

From the very first studies, people like Henri Laborit and Jean Delay were impressed by the fact that, under the influence of chlorpromazine, people seemed to pay little heed to their environment, and to be perceptually indifferent, even though their sensory abilities were fully intact and they were awake. In this way the drugs differ from barbiturates, which reduce one's interest in his environment only in proportion to their tendency to put one to sleep. The British psychopharmacologist Philip Bradley was able to pin this down in elegant fashion using experimental animals. He recorded the brain waves (electroencephalogram) and observed the behavior of cats. He could produce arousal, as monitored by the brain waves or the animal's overt behavior, either by direct stimulation of the brain stem, which contains a well-known arousal system, or by a sensory stimulus such as a clicking noise. Barbiturates affect the brain stem arousal system directly, since in very small doses they block the arousal normally produced by brain stem stimulation or by the click. Chlorpromazine on the other hand had no effect upon arousal that had been elicited by brain stem stimulation. However, in very low doses it interfered with arousal in response to the clicking noise.

Bradley concluded that barbiturates owe their sedating and sleep-inducing actions to a direct depression of the arousal system in the brain stem, which scientists believe to play a major role in regulating sleep–wakefulness. Phenothiazines don't act that way. Chlorpromazine appears to affect arousal by interfering with the ability of sensory stimuli to "get through." Schizophrenics, of course, are overloaded with their environment, so much so that they have retreated far behind the defense lines of their psyches. Reasoning from Dr. Bradley's findings, one can readily think of the phenothiazines as "turning off" the environmental bombardment, making the world less terrifying and an easier place with which to cope.

3

Psychedelicrazy

Many people have the impression that psychedelic drugs are a discovery of the 1960s. For them, the primary explorer and discoverer is Timothy Leary, who in the early 1960s began to administer psilocybin and later LSD to graduate students at Harvard University. But Timothy Leary is only the popularizer. Psychedelic drugs have a long and rich history. Many years before Columbus discovered America, Aztec Indians in Mexico were utilizing the peyote plant, whose active ingredient is mescaline, as part of their religious ceremonies. Preparations akin to hashish and marijuana, which are lumped together with psychedelic drugs by many writers, were in use in India over a thousand years ago. Systematic scientific experimentation with well-characterized chemical forms of such substances had even been under way before the turn of the twentieth century. LSD, the relative newcomer among the psychedelic agents, was synthesized by Albert Hofmann at the Sandoz Drug Company in Switzerland in 1938. In 1943 he accidentally discovered its incredible effects on the mind. So, in fact, psychedelic drugs had been extensively studied well before Timothy Leary himself had ever popped a pill of LSD.

Why are psychedelic drugs so indelibly associated with the sixth decade of the twentieth century? What happened in the 1960s to bring them to the fore? Of course the simplest answer is that in the 1960s the general public became aware of these compounds. For years mescaline and a variety of other psychedelic compounds were listed in the catalogues of many chemical supply houses, where they could be purchased at ridiculously low prices and with no special identification or registration of the buyer. But, except for psychopharmacologists, no one paid much heed.

However, it is not enough simply to say that in the 1960s psychedelics caught the public's imagination. There had been enough descriptions of the remarkable properties of these chemicals, descriptions framed for the general public, that, were the climate right, the compounds could readily have attained wide popularity much earlier. The key element is "climate"; that is, the context in which the drugs were used and their significance to the user. In the 1960s, psychedelic drugs represented a "turned on, tuned in, drop out" escape from a world filled with hypocritical values, Vietnamese wars, and so on. For the ancient Aztec Indians, and still for several thousand members of the Native American Church of the Southwestern United States, psychedelic drugs are a religious sacrament. To some medical researchers, they are a means of inducing an experimental form of schizophrenia.

What Are They?

The psychedelic drugs are a group of compounds of widely varying chemical structures, which all share the ability to produce a strikingly similar set of profound subjective experiences. They have been called many names, such as hallucinogenic, psychotomimetic, psychedelic, psychodysleptic, psychosomimetic, psychotogenic and phantastica. The choice depends on the context in which the writer wishes to view the drugs. If one is interested in analyzing the nature of sensory perception and is intrigued by the drug-induced perceptual distortions, then "hallucinogenic" might seem an appropriate term. For those who wish to plumb the fathoms of their innermost minds, then the drugs become "psychedelic," which means mind-manifesting or mind-expanding. And those who wonder whether the LSD state might teach them something about the world of the schizophrenic are dealing with "psychotomimetic" or "psychotogenic" agents.

One of the most remarkable facets of the psychedelic drugs is the fact that, although they don't resemble one another very much in their molecular structures, they do have closely related subjective effects. LSD is a complex multiringed chemical (see appendix) which bears little resemblance to mescaline; yet, except for certain nuances, the changes in perception and cognition brought about by the two drugs are virtually indistinguishable. By contrast, mescaline is a close chemical relative of amphetamine. However, amphetamine, though it may cause psychosis if taken in large enough doses, never gives rise to anything resembling a psychedelic experience. There are a whole host of derivatives of mescaline whose chemical structure includes part of the amphetamine molecule. All of these are mainly psychedelic drugs, whose effects are quite unlike those of amphetamine, although some produce in the user a little bit of the amphetaminelike central stimulant high.

The Psychedelic Experience

What usually happens to an individual under the influence of a psychedelic drug? Of course, the variety of psychedelic experiences is as great as human nature itself. Everything is possible, from a complete absence of effects in psychologically unsophisticated subjects who are trying to avoid the experience, up to and including a complete loss of identity, a peculiar and ineffable feeling that one's self has merged with the totality of the universe, or a spiritual experience as profound as the "discovery of God" by great religious leaders. Despite the potential variations of experience in any given psychedelic session, there are some typical events.

A moderate dose of LSD (about 100–200 micrograms), such as I consumed once about ten years ago, produces few discernible effects for the first thirty minutes or so. At this time there might be slight nausea, which is rarely severe enough to cause vomiting. Soon, the sensory effects begin. Objects in the visual field may take on a purplish tinge, or seen vaguely outlined. Everything perceived—colors, textures, lines—attain a beauty and richness never seen before. Perception seems to be so incisive that the individual pores in your skin almost stand out and clamor for recognition. You may feel that your visual powers penetrate other people to plumb their secret selves. Contours of objects may become distorted much as in the late paintings of Van Gogh. These distortions often reflect the feelings and wishes of the individual. For instance, if you look at your hand and focus upon the thumb, the thumb may proceed to swell, undulate, and even begin moving toward you in a menacing fashion.

The sense of time changes dramatically. A minute may seem like an hour, a week like all eternity. One day ago feels so long past that it might as well have existed only in some prior life. Since the present seems to drag on to infinity, the very concept of "future" loses any meaning. The time changes result from a speeding up of mental processes. Since one's perceptions and feelings are so heightened that they are intensively recording every instant, one feels that more events are transpiring per unit of time; or, viewed differently, time slows down.

Similarly, distances change. Flicking one's finger seems like hurling it across the room, and walking across the room is like traversing the corners of the universe. Presumably, as a consequence of the alterations in the perception of time and distance, there occurs the remarkable phenomenon of synesthesia. Synesthesia is like a transmutation of the senses. The subject may *see* sounds or *hear* colors. When I was under the influence of LSD and someone in the room clapped their hands, I could, or thought I could, see the sound waves undulate before me. I don't know what would happen in this circumstance with a subject who has never studied high school physics.

Closing one's eyes often produces remarkable visions filled with vivid and persistent eidetic imagery. For instance, one of the subjects studied by Jean Houston, a prominent researcher with psychedelic drugs, reported seeing the following sequences when he closed his eyes: "There are snakes, alligators, dragons, beautiful reptiles. They are lying at the bottom of a kind of sea, but I don't think it is water. At the edges of this place where they are, there are tigers walking along the shore. Up on the beach all kinds of wild orgies are going on. Lots of sex. People getting drunk, and tigers eating people. Tigers getting drunk on blood, and then slaughtering one another."

At the stage in which sensory effects predominate, the subject is so enmeshed in the rich and varied world about him that he takes little account of any changes in his sense of self, or at least these are not reported during the initial phases with the drug. The only "psychological" change noticed early on is uncontrolled giggling; however, as one becomes accustomed, as much as that is possible, to the riotous changes in sensation, then psychological influences become apparent. One major type of change is self-reflection. One becomes aware of thoughts and feelings long hidden beneath the surface, forgotten and/or repressed. Some enthusiasts even claim that psychedelic drugs accomplish in a period of hours what Freud set forth as the task of a complete psychoanalytic treatment regimen of several years, namely to "make conscious the unconscious."

Frequently, the insights which people gain as to their true motives and attitudes toward important persons in their lives while under the influence of LSD are precise and valid insights. Just as sensory processing of information is enhanced, so what psychoanalysts call "free association" races along under the influence of the drug and its scope is greatly extended. Such insights can have valuable psychotherapeutic influence upon the drug user for long periods after having taken the drug. On the other hand, if the setting is not quite right, or the subject is anxious, the psychedelic drug session evolves into a "bad trip." Recollections of long-dormant feelings may be frightening and precipitate neurotic or even psychotic symptoms.

A similar capacity for both good and bad arises in the next phase. Though some people may never go beyond the dredging up of earlier attitudes about life, in others this reflecting upon the relation of self and the world goes deeper and deeper until it reaches a level at which self and world fuse. This is the mystical–spiritual aspect of the drug experience. It is indescribable. For how can anyone verbalize a merging of his being with the totality of the universe? How do you put into words the feeling that "all is one," "I am of the all," "I am no longer"? One's skin ceases to be a boundary between self and other. This state is very much like that experienced by Hindu and Christian mystics. It can bring with it a profound sense of serenity and peaceful contemplation, with attendant love toward all one's fellow men.

On the other hand, what we have just described is essentially a loss of self-identity—a dissolving of ego boundaries. For many people, the sense of self is already somewhat tenuous. For such individuals with weak ego boundaries, as well as for uptight, rigid people who demand that their world be familiar and well-ordered, these changes are intolerable. As we discussed earlier, the fragmentation of the ego is what gives rise to panic in schizophrenic patients. In many people under the influence of psychedelic drugs, the panic which follows upon realization that the subject doesn't know who he is, where he is, or what has come of his world, this panic is no less terrifying than that known to acute schizophrenics. It is in such drug-induced panic states that people have jumped from windows to their death or themselves commited homicide. While we know a little about factors in the environment which are conducive to "good trips" as opposed to bad ones, one can never reliably predict whether a given individual will or will not undergo such a terrifying experience.

Different Drugs

So it goes with LSD. Although the sequence of events during a session with LSD are fairly similar to those occurring with other psychedelic drugs, there are certain nuances of differences among the various compounds. The effects of a moderate dose of LSD will last for about eight hours. Though the subject may be a little shaky the next day, he does not usually notice any residual drug effects. Occasionally, if he was a victim of a particularly severe "bad trip," there may be some perceptual changes intermittently for a day or two. Of course, if the drug precipitates an acute psychotic breakdown, a happily uncommon event, then he will be gravely ill for a variable period of a few days to years. In this case, however, the psychosis will be more a reflection of his own peculiar mental make-up, and not of the drug which will have served only as a precipitant.

The various psychedelic drugs differ somewhat in their effects. Some of these differences may provide clues as to the fundamental actions of these drugs on the mind. DOM, frequently referred to by drug users as "STP," when used in fairly high doses can be longer lasting. Often typical psychedelic effects continue into the next day. DOM was first synthesized by Dr. Alexander Shulgin, one of the most eminent chemists in the synthetic development of new psychedelic agents, as an analogue of mescaline which would not be as readily degraded in the body and, hence, might be active at lower doses. Indeed, DOM is fifty to 100 times more potent than mescaline, and, because it is not as readily broken down, it persists longer in the body, which accounts for its ability to produce symptoms for a longer period than LSD or mescaline. Chemically, DOM is something of a cross between mescaline and amphetamine. Many users have reported that DOM, besides causing typical psychedelic effects, also elicits some of the jitteriness and enhanced alertness associated normally with amphetamines. However, because all psychedelic drugs are to a certain extent central stimulants, it is difficult to be sure whether the psychological effects of DOM incorporate those of amphetamines as well as those of conventional psychedelic drugs.

Mescaline is somewhat longer acting than LSD; its effects persist for about twelve hours. Psychedelic experiences with mescaline tend to be smoother, with less anxiety than occurs with LSD. Under the influence of mescaline users generally focus more upon the sensual, perceptual effects. They become more entranced with their surroundings, often for the total duration of the drug session, and spend less time in introspection than they would with LSD.

Mescaline and its chemical relative, DOM, differ greatly in molecular layout from LSD. Psilocybin and dimethyltryptamine (called DMT by users), by contrast, are fairly similar though less complex in their chemical structure to LSD. The general complexion of the effects elicited by psilocybin and DMT are very much like those of LSD. Psilocybin lasts for a shorter period of time than LSD—about four hours—and DMT acts for an even more dramatically brief period. From start to finish the complete sequence consumes only forty-five minutes to an hour. DMT is spoken of as "the business man's luncheon psychedelic," since, when the hour is up, restitution to normality is usually complete. Almost all psychedelic drugs can be taken by mouth. However, DMT appears to be destroyed in the stomach or in the intestines and so must be given by injection or by inhalation ("snorting"). Of course, either injection or inhalation will produce effects more rapidly than swallowing a pill, so that DMT has become widely hailed for its extraordinarily abrupt onset, commonly referred to as a "mind explosion."

MDA is another mescaline–amphetamine derivative with certain remarkable features. It is reputed, on good authority, to produce only "good trips." How can it be that a psychedelic drug could specialize only in pleasant experiences? Presumably the drugs trigger some psychological action which is responsible for the "badness" of some trips, an action which MDA apparently lacks. If we only knew what biochemical changes in the brain were responsible for the goodness or badness of drug experiences, we might be in a position to produce new drugs which would be the ultimate in enhancing self-awareness, but always evoking happy experiences.

What do drug users describe about the MDA experience which might account for its characteristically pleasant effects? Among those I have interviewed, the most frequent feature which might account for the difference between MDA and LSD is that, unlike LSD, MDA rarely provokes intense anxiety. Under the influence of LSD, users maintain that they feel pushed, driven to plumb the depths of their inner self. The drug won't let them alone until they have slashed through every inch of their psyche, relentlessly examining and reexamining every feeling and memory. By contrast, the MDA experience just "happens," and there is no pressure to deal with any particular emotional facet. The user tunes in whatever part of his inner or outer world that he chooses.

MDA differs in yet another way from the other psychedelic drugs. At most doses there are few, if any, perceptual disturbances. It is possible to obtain vivid sensory images if one closes his eyes and searches. However, with eyes open, the perceived environment is hardly altered. Along with the lessened anxiety and perceptual changes, and perhaps because of them, there seems to be less of a tendency to become psychotic with MDA. By psychotic, I mean that the thinking processes of the individual are so different from those of other people that most would judge him to have "lost contact with reality." With LSD, as soon as you reach doses which will consistently produce any effects in subjects, the behavior of the user changes so strikingly that he would be generally judged psychotic; hence, LSD is a psychotomimetic drug. At equivalent doses MDA is not really psychotomimetic, although it could be at higher doses.

These features of MDA are exaggerated even more in another mescaline–amphetamine analogue, DOET. This drug differs only in a minor way from DOM and, like DOM, was synthesized by Alexander Shulgin as part of his program to develop more and more potent psychedelic agents. In terms of the minimal dose necessary to elicit any subjective effects, DOET is probably twice as potent as DOM. However, Drs. Louis Faillace, Herbert

Weingartner, and myself, in our studies of this drug's actions in non–mental patients at Johns Hopkins Hospital, found that it differed in several important ways from DOM. With DOM, when we doubled the minimal dose which could be detected at all by our subjects, we began to see clearcut psychotomimetic–hallucinogenic effects. By contrast, even when DOET was fed in amounts five times greater than the minimal detectable quantity, there was no evidence of psychotomimetric or hallucinogenic changes. Subjects invariably reported a feeling of enhanced self-awareness. They could describe feelings which they recognized to be valid but which were normally "just below the surface." They also tended to feel relaxed, and a little happier than they had reason to be, more euphoric, perhaps as they would when smoking marijuana.

As an "active" placebo, we had compared the effects of DOET to those of amphetamines. The differences which subjects reported between the two drugs were impressive. One subject described it this way: "[Under the influence of DOET] I am more likely to have interesting or new associations of ideas. I was able to associate images with my thoughts better today. The other drug [amphetamine] just helped concentration but wasn't relaxing and didn't help me to associate at all except in a very limited sense. It didn't help spontaneous notions to come in. In fact it rather kept them out . . . . You can make me giggle if you want . . . A number of things are closer to the surface than they normally would be . . . I was tremendously suggestible today. I could be pushed in a lot of directions."

The differences in the subtleties of effects produced by drugs like MDA and DOET from those produced by

LSD may have several important implications. For instance, a drug like DOET might be useful in facilitating psychotherapy. Under its influence, patients might have more ready access to their strongest, most deeply hidden feelings. LSD also "makes conscious the unconscious" and has been tried out as an aid in psychotherapy. The hope was that LSD would enable rigid, obsessional people to "loosen up" and express their deeper, usually guarded feelings. But with LSD, the changes in perception and the psychotomimetic effects interfere. How can a patient focus on his psychotherapy when he is constantly being distracted by the transformed world that he beholds around him and when his thinking processes are decidedly askew? A drug like DOET, on the other hand, can also make latent feelings accessible, but the patient has full command of his mental faculties and can direct all his energies toward therapy.

Over and above their therapeutic potential, drugs like MDA and DOET may teach us something quite important about how psychedelic drugs act. If, with some drugs, the "mind manifesting" actions appear at the same doses as the psychotomimetic–hallucinogenic alterations, while in other drugs these effects are separable, one might postulate that these are separate and distinct actions of the drugs. Perhaps we should be searching in the brain for two discrete places where psychedelic drugs might act. One would be the true "psychedelic" locus, which mediates access to varied thoughts and feelings and hence regulates the level of self-awareness. The other, the hallucinogenic–psychotomimetic area, might determine the distortion of perception and would be responsible for the psychotomimetic "break from reality."

Marijuana

Where does marijuana fit in? Some people look upon marijuana as a minor psychedelic agent. They feel that it does the same things as conventional psychedelic drugs but is much weaker. Marijuana effects are much like those of DOET. Subjects feel a little euphoric. Everything they hear, see, smell, or taste is more vivid and occasionally distorted. Some users feel that marijuana puts them in close contact with their private feelings. With very potent preparations of marijuana, such as those that come from certain parts of Mexico, Thailand, or Vietnam, or with hashish, a concentrated form of marijuana which is about ten times as active as most marijuana used in the United States, frankly hallucinogenic and psychotomimetic effects are common.

A number of eminent writers in the nineteenth century became greatly interested in hashish. They even formed clubs devoted to its use, and in this way probably deserve the credit for first introducing the psychedelic experience to Western culture. They must have been utilizing fairly powerful hashish as their experiences remind one of typical LSD sessions.

The French writer Théophile Gautier described changes in perception and distortions which were sufficiently like those of LSD that one would label hashish "hallucinogenic": "[B]y some strange miracle, after a few moments of rapt contemplation I merged into the object of my gaze, and I myself became that object." Existence of time and distance was enormously altered. ". . . I rose with great difficulty and headed toward the door of the drawing room. My progress was painfully slow, for an unknown force made me take one step backward for every three steps forward. In my reckoning it took me ten years to reach the door . . . I reached the adjoining room. Its dimensions had changed beyond recognition; it stretched on and on without end. A light that glimmered at the far side of the room seemed as remote as a fixed star." At the depth of his intoxication, Gautier was clearly psychotic: "[A]t this point the intoxication completely overpowered me; I went stark mad. [I perceived that my companion appeared to have] somersaulted to the ceiling shrieking 'you fool I gave you back your head but I scooped the brains out first.'"

The American writer Bayard Taylor, during his years in Damascus, came into contact with hashish, and in 1855 wrote about it describing his loss of contact with reality:

> I tore open my vest, placed my hand over the spot, and tried to count the pulsations; but there were two hearts, one beating at the rate of 1000 beats a minute, and the other with a slow, dull motion. My throat, I felt, was filled to the brim with blood, and streams of blood were pouring from my ears. I felt them gushing warm down my cheeks and neck . . . My body seemed to shrink and grow rigid as I wrestled with the demon and my face to become wild, lean and haggard. . . . Oh horrors! The flesh had fallen from my bones, and it was a skeleton head that I carried on my shoulders . . . I was sinking deeper and deeper into a pit of unutterable agony and despair. . . . Every effort to preserve my reason was accompanied by a pang of mortal fear, lest what I now experienced was insanity, and would hold mastery over me forever. The thought of death, which also haunted me, was far less bitter than this dread.

Marijuana can enhance self-awareness. Although potent forms of the drug can be psychotomimetic and hallucinogenic, is it to be classed with the psychedelic drugs? We cannot reason from any similarities in chem-

ical structure. The molecular form of tetrahydrocan-
nabinol, the active ingredient of marijuana and hashish,
doesn't resemble any of the psychedelic drugs; in fact, it
does not resemble any of the drugs known to man.

Moreover, despite their similarities, the psychological effects of marijuana can be differentiated from those
of the psychedelic drugs. A number of investigators,
especially Dr. Harris Isbell at the University of Kentucky,
have compared the symptoms elicited by psychedelic
drugs and those of marijuana or THC. Even though
psychedelic drugs differ in the subtleties of their effects,
they tend to act more like each other than like marijuana. Unlike psychedelic drugs, which dramatically
heighten one's state of alertness, marijuana is something of a soporific. Smokers want to sleep after a pot
session. In fact, in nineteenth-century medical practice,
marijuana was widely prescribed as a sedative and
sleeping medication. Also, unlike psychedelics marijuana greatly stimulates appetite. In India it is prescribed as a tonic to fatten up skinny children. Thus,
whether to include marijuana in the same class as
psychedelic drugs is still an open question.

Model Psychoses

The widespread interest in psychedelic drugs on the
part of the general public throughout the world seems
to stem from their potential for pointing toward a new
way of experiencing the universe, a hitherto unsus-
pected face of mental life, a novel spiritualism to replace
the vanishing faith in traditional religion. However, more
than a decade before Timothy Leary began proselytizing
and spreading the "word" to millions of people, scien-

tists and psychiatrists were fascinated with psychedelic drugs for very different reasons. They sought in these agents tools to elicit model psychoses which might mimic the symptoms of schizophrenia.

The idea is simple and can be approached in at least two straightforward ways. If the symptoms produced by drugs like LSD resemble those of schizophrenia closely and meaningfully, then all we need to do is to find out just how LSD does its thing within the brain, and we have for ourselves a reasonable guess as to what might be the malfunction in schizophrenia. The second approach holds that the bodies of schizophrenics might produce a toxic substance which resembles psychedelic agents.

Interest in this latter view was spurred on by a provocative paper published in 1952 by two British psychiatrists, Humphrey Osmond and John Smythies. They described the rationale behind the model psychosis approach to studies of schizophrenia and then reported an observation by a chemist colleague of theirs, Dr. Harley-Mason. All Harley-Mason did was to point out to Osmond and Smythies the impressive chemical similarity between adrenaline (the chemical secretion of the adrenal gland which accounts for "fight and flight" reactions of the body under stress) and the mescaline molecule. If the body could transform adrenaline into something resembling mescaline, here would be the sought for schizophrenia-causing toxin.

What seemed like the answer to the fondest hopes of Osmond and Smythies was soon forthcoming. Dr. Abram Hoffer in Saskatchewan reported on a remarkable derivative of adrenaline which he claimed to find in the body fluids of schizophrenics. When solutions of adrenaline are left to stand at room temperature for a brief period they turn pink. What has happened is that the adrenaline is oxidized (combines with oxygen from the air) to something called adrenochrome, which has an intense red color. Hoffer reported two spectacular breakthroughs. First, he could detect adrenochrome in the blood and urine of a large number of schizophrenics but not in most nonschizophrenic individuals. How might this be related to their illness? He also claimed that, when administered to normal human subjects, adrenochrome evoked a psychedelic sort of experience which resembled schizophrenia even more than typical LSD effects. Under the influence of adrenochrome, his volunteers felt strangely unreal, depersonalized, and out of emotional contact with other people, hence withdrawn and autistic. It would seem that the millennium of psychiatry had arrived.

Needless to say, investigators all over the world hastened to follow up these major breakthroughs. What they found out teaches a bitter but important lesson for all psychiatric investigators. Let not thy enthusiasm carry thee away! When rigorous chemical measurements of adrenochrome were performed, it became quite clear that adrenochrome is not present in anyone's blood, schizophrenic or nonschizophrenic. Perhaps without even being aware of it, in their eagerness to prove the adrenochrome theory of schizophrenia, Hoffer and his technicians were simply letting the schizophrenic samples stand on the laboratory bench longer than the nonschizophrenic samples, with the result that adrenaline was converted to adrenochrome. Whatever the reasons, there is little doubt that adrenochrome is not a unique chemical constituent in the bodies of schizophrenics.

Numerous chemists have reexamined the question again and again, hoping that there might have been some tinge of truth in Hoffer's observations, but they could find none. What about adrenochrome as a psychedelic drug? It should be quite simple to devise experiments to verify these findings. All one needs are human volunteers and a supply of adrenochrome, a reasonably cheap chemical. Accordingly, psychiatric investigators all over the world soon were exploring the purported psychedelic actions of adrenochrome. But no one could find any. The drug was no more active than tap water. What Hoffer seems to have observed was a simple placebo effect. All his subjects knew that they were receiving adrenochrome, a drug which was supposed to make them a little bit schizophrenic. Hoffer never compared adrenochrome with a placebo, in a way that the subjects would not know when they were getting placebo and when adrenochrome was the drug. Accordingly, Hoffer's breakthrough was no more than another demonstration of the extraordinary power of suggestion.

Disillusionment, Distrust

After the adrenochrome fiasco, psychiatrists became disillusioned and immensely skeptical about the drug-induced model psychosis approach to schizophrenia. They reexamined just how much psychedelic drug effects resemble those of schizophrenic patients. The initial enthusiasm had been sparked by a simpleminded notion that the drugs do produce psychosis and do produce hallucinations, both major characteristics of schizophrenia. Now psychiatrists began to examine more critically details of the similarities and differences between schizophrenic symptoms and psychedelic drug effects. One must bear in mind that all sorts of drugs can evoke psychosis and hallucinations at high enough doses. Bromide, used widely fifty years ago as a sedative, provides an example. When the drug is ingested for over a month, it accumulates in the body, and at a certain point bromide psychosis, complete with hallucinations and delusions, supervenes. The bromide psychosis is a typical organic brain dysfunction, with confusion, disorientation, and delirium. In this way it differs from the psychedelic drugs, whose effects, like the symptoms of schizophrenia, occur in a setting of clear consciousness. Indeed with LSD, subjects are hyperalert and remember every detail of their drug session. Still, there are marked differences between psychedelic drug experiences and schizophrenia.

Leo Hollister, one of the more skeptical investigators, approached the question in a straightforward fashion. He asked a group of mental health professionals to listen to tape-recorded interviews conducted either with schizophrenic or with normal subjects under the influence of psychedelic drugs and guess which were which. There were virtually no mistakes. The raters were consummately accurate in differentiating schizophrenia from the effects of psychedelic drugs. Hollister summarized what a number of the raters considered the characteristic difference between the groups "in the schizophrenics the primary disturbance was in thinking [and by this was meant something far more subtle than incoherence], while the drug subjects' disturbance was in perceptions." Thus, even though thinking and feeling are altered by psychedelic drugs, the changes are very different, apparently less thoroughgoing than those of the schizophrenic.

Another way of getting at the same question is to give LSD to schizophrenics and to see how they fare. If the drug accentuates their schizophrenic symptoms, one might look on it as a schizophrenia-mimicking agent. When numerous investigators have treated schizophrenic subjects with LSD, they have been impressed by the fact that the drug did not simply worsen the schizophrenia. It produced the typical spectrum of psychedelic actions, which were clearly different from the schizophrenic symptoms. Moreover, the patients themselves were able to detect and describe the differences between the drug's actions and their own illness.

Even though schizophrenics hallucinate and subjects under the influence of psychedelic drugs hallucinate, one must be wary about likening the two situations. The perceptual distortions elicited by LSD tend to be primarily visual, while schizophrenic hallucinations are usually auditory and involve voices. Psychiatrist Irwin Feinberg analyzed schizophrenic and LSD-induced hallucinations in great detail. Even the visual hallucinations of schizophrenics differ in important ways from those induced by psychedelic drugs. For instance, in schizophrenia, visual hallucinations appear suddenly and without warning, while those of mescaline and LSD are

> ... heralded by unformed visual sensations, simple geometric figures, and alterations of color, size, shape, movement and number. Furthermore, schizophrenic hallucinations may be superimposed on a visual environment that appears otherwise normal, or, more rarely, they may appear with the remainder of the environment excluded. The drugs produce diffuse distortions of the existing visual world. Schizophrenic hallucinations are generally seen with the eyes open; those of mescaline and LSD are more readily seen with the eyes closed or in darkened surroundings.

As contrasts between psychedelic drug and schizophrenic psychoses accumulated, researchers became more and more disillusioned with the notion that LSD elicits a model schizophrenia. The more sophisticated among them did not altogether reject the model psychosis concept but felt that a more subtle formulation would be necessary. There are several reasons for not discounting outright a relationship between psychedelic drug psychosis and schizophrenia. In comparing the two conditions, one ought not really expect to find perfect congruity. Remember that the individual swallowing an LSD tablet has many years of normal emotional functioning in the world behind him. Moreover, he knows that whatever happens to him during the drug session will only be temporary, that there is nothing to fear. By contrast, a schizophrenic patient has been interacting within his environment in an aberrant way, probably since he was a small child. He has never known emotional security. Worst of all, he recognizes that his psychosis is not a trivial matter of eight hours' duration. By the time most schizophrenics reach the clutches of the experimenter, they have been experiencing the pangs of their illness for substantial periods, at least months and often years.

Perhaps a better analogy between psychedelic drug psychosis and schizophrenia would be made if one administered a hefty dose of LSD four times a day every day for three months. How would subjects think and experience the world under those conditions? Of course such an experiment is out of the question. The best we can do is to study the limited number of very heavy, chronic uses of psychedelic drugs, the "acid heads." Interestingly, psychological evaluation of these people suggests that they are somewhat out of touch with reality. Their thinking patterns are vague and characterized by somewhat loose associations. Like many early schizophrenics, they often center their lives about magical, astrological, and pseudoreligious movements. However, few of these individuals are frankly schizophrenic. Moreover, it is difficult to be sure that their psychological hangups have been *caused* by the drug. Remember, these are people who have chosen for themselves a life of heavy drug use, estranged from everyday society. Perhaps they would behave and think in this subtly disturbed fashion even if they had not been heavy users of the drugs.

Psychedelia

Because of the new skepticism toward psychedelic drugs as tools to unravel the mysteries of schizophrenia, the focus of interest shifted from their hallucinogenic effects to their mind-expanding psychedelic properties. Interestingly, the same sequence of events usually transpires within a given psychedelic drug session. First interest centers on perceptual changes and "minor" mental manifestations, to be followed by the more profound introspective psychedelic concerns. Humphrey Osmond introduced the scientific community to this new approach at a meeting of the New York Academy of Sciences where he coined the word "psychedelic." The conference was entitled the "Pharmacology of Psychotomimetic . . . Drugs," which irked Osmond. For, he argued,

> If mimicking mental illness were the main characteristic of these agents, 'psychotomimetic' would indeed be a suitable generic term. It is true that they do so, but they do much more. Why are we always preoccupied with the pathological, the negative? Is health only the lack of sickness? Is good merely the absence of evil? Is pathology the only

yardstick? Must we ape Freud's gloomier moods that persuaded him that a happy man is a self-deceiver evading the heartache for which there is no anodyne? Is not a child infinitely potential rather than polymorphously perverse?

Accordingly, he attempted to evolve a new name to emphasize the positive aspects of the drugs: "I have tried to find an appropriate name for the agents under discussion: a name that will include the concepts of enriching the mind and enlarging the vision . . . my choice, because it is clear, euphonious, and uncontaminated by other associations, is psychedelic, mind-manifesting."

Many people have written of their experiences with psychedelic drugs. Few have done so with such clarity as Aldous Huxley, who wrote a short book, *The Doors of Perception*, describing his impressions of the day he ingested mescaline. The psychedelic quality of events lived through under the influence of a drug like mescaline or LSD is difficult to put into words. Far more impressive than simple distortions of objects impressed upon the sense organs is the way in which the viewer is entranced with the very being of the object perceived and with its relation to his own self and of his self to the universe.

Huxley recognized this an hour and a half after ingesting the pill of mescaline, when he was gazing upon a small glass vase containing three flowers. He did not see the flowers as particularly distorted. Instead something more remarkable was happening. "I was not looking now at an unusual flower arrangement. I was seeing what Adam had seen on the morning of his creation—the miracle, moment by moment, of naked existence." When asked by someone "is it agreeable," he responded,

. . . neither agreeable or disagreeable, it just *is* . . . wasn't that the word Meister Eckhart [a famous Christian mystic] liked to use? Is-ness. The being of platonic philosophy—except that Plato seems to have made the enormous, the grotesque mistake of separating Being from Becoming . . . an identifying with the mathematical abstraction of the Idea. He could never, poor fellow, have seen a bunch of flowers shining with their own inner light and all but quivering under the pressure of the significance with which they were charged; could never have perceived that what a rose, an iris, carnation so intensely signified was nothing more, and nothing less, than what they were—a transience that was yet eternal life, a perpetual perishing that was at the same time pure Being, a bundle of minute, unique particulars in which, by some unspeakable and yet self-evident paradox, was to be seen the divine source of all existence.

Huxley even suggested a way in which the changes in the sense of time and space which are elicited by psychedelic drugs might be a product of this peculiar concern with Being:

[P]lace and distance cease to be of much interest. The mind does its perceiving in terms of intensity of existence, profundity of significance, relationships within a pattern. I saw the books but was not at all concerned with their positions in space . . . What impressed itself on my mind was the fact that all of them glowed with living light and in some the glory was more manifest than in others . . . the mind was primarily concerned, not with measures and locations, but with being and meaning.

Huxley felt that his fixation upon the essence and existence of objects that he perceived might underlie the mystical experience of the merging of self with the environment, indeed with the universe.

The legs, for example, of that chair—how miraculous their tubularity, how supernatural their polished smoothness! I spent several minutes—or was it several centuries?—not merely gazing at those bamboo legs, but actually *being* them—or rather being myself in them; or, to be still more accurate (for "I" was not involved in the case—nor in a certain sense were "they") being my not-self in the not-self which was the chair.

It was clearly the "psychedelic" character of LSD effects which accounted for Timothy Leary's fascination with the drug and which started him on the path of proselytizing American youth, an expedition to "turn on the world." The movement took on full definition with the emergence of the hippies in San Francisco's Haight-Ashbury district, a self-contained culture, complete with prescribed uniform, diet, and music.

The notion that psychedelic drugs elicit a profound change in one's sense of being also gave rise to attempts to utilize profound psychedelic experiences as a means of therapy for patients with a variety of disabilities, particularly alcoholism. The rationale is simply that the overwhelming changes in self-identity elicited by the drug can be utilized, if directed by a skilled psychotherapist, to produce a change in the patient's life style. There is something about the sensation of at-oneness with the universe which makes all petty concerns seem silly and sparks one to want to live a more noble life. Huxley describes it this way "When we feel ourselves to be sole heirs of the universe when 'the sea flows in our veins . . . and the stars are our jewels,' when all things are perceived as infinite and holy, what motive can we have for covetousness or self-assertion, for the pursuit of power or the drearier forms of pleasure."

There have been many reports of spectacular improvement in the behavior of patients who have undergone a profound psychedelic experience with LSD. With alcoholics, such improvement is readily measured by determining if the patient no longer drinks, and for how long he remains abstinent. Despite the simplicity of assessing the effectiveness of psychedelic drug therapy with alcoholics, the question of the efficacy of this treatment, like so many other questions with psychedelic drugs, has remained confusing and controversial.

In the psychedelic form of treatment, patients receive extensive psychotherapeutic preparation prior to the drug session. Some researchers, attempting to find out what role this pre-drug "coaching" played in the therapeutic response to LSD, provided one group with such intensive psychotherapy and with no LSD, while the other group received both psychotherapeutic preparation and the drug. It turned out that there was no difference between the subsequent fate of the two groups. Both groups of patients became abstinent and described their "conversion" to a new life with enthusiasm bordering on ecstasy. However, within six months after the end of the treatment, almost all had returned to his old habits of heavy drinking.

Another therapeutic effort with LSD involved administering it to terminal cancer patients. In initial studies it seemed as if the psychedelic experience, like many mystical experiences, enabled some patients to meet their death with equanimity. One investigator reported that patients treated with LSD required much lower doses of narcotic painkillers. Even if the number of patients who could benefit from this treatment are few, it would seem immensely worthwhile. Certainly with dying patients there would be little concern about abuse of the drugs.

*A New Link of Psychedelic Drugs
and Schizophrenia*

Whether or not psychedelic drugs are effective therapy for any type of emotional maladjustment, one can hardly deny the extraordinary impact of the true psychedelic experience. Perhaps, aside from the utility of these drugs in therapy, the awesome, unworldly, mystical nature of the psychedelic experience may convey valuable lessons about certain aspects of mental illness, lessons which are possibly more useful than the model psychosis concept.

The true psychedelic experience is somewhat reminiscent of the "primary delusions" of incipient schizophrenics. Early in their disease numerous patients feel overwhelmed by remarkable inner happenings. Unlike their later illness, these initial events can be quite pleasant. The American psychiatrists Malcolm Bowers and Daniel X. Freedman reviewed a number of case histories of schizophrenics and were impressed by what sounded very much like psychedelic experiences in the early, acute phases of the schizophrenic breakdown. The uncanny sensation of extraordinary clarity, seeing into the essences and beings of all objects, is evident in a number of their patients.

One of them described how the world suddenly became "a completely wonderful place . . . I began to experience goodness and love for the first time." Another patient reported:

Before last week I was quite closed about my emotions; then finally I owned up to them with another person. I began to speak without thinking beforehand and what came out showed an awareness of human beings and God. I could feel deeply about other people. I felt connected. The side which had been suppressing emotions did not seem to be the real one. I was in a higher and higher state of exhilaration and awareness. Things people said had hidden meaning. They said things that applied to life. Everything that was real seemed to make sense. I had a great awareness of life, truth, and God. I went to church and suddenly all parts of the service made sense. My senses were sharpened. I became fascinated by the little insignificant things around me. There was an additional awareness of the world that would do artists, architects, and painters good.

A feeling of very special significance in small events and objects, which will later crystalize into delusions, is evident in another of the patients of Bowers and Freedman:

Thoughts spun around in my head and everything—objects, sound, events—took on special meaning for me. I felt like I was putting the pieces of a puzzle together. Childhood feelings began to come back, as symbols and bits from past conversations went through my head. The word *religious* and other words from other past conversations . . . came back to me during this week . . . I increasingly began to feel that I was experiencing something like mystical revelations . . . At the gas station the men smiled at me with twinkles in their eyes, and I felt very good. I saw smiling men's faces in the sky and the stars twinkling in their eyes. I felt better than I ever had in my life.

The extraordinary vividness of sensations which is characteristic of all psychedelic drugs was emphasized by another patient, who reported, "My senses were sharpened, sounds were more intense, and I could see with greater clarity, everything seemed very clear to me. Even my sense of taste seemed more acute."

Numerous schizophrenics have published accounts of their illness, some of which are quite eloquent. Ms.

Norma McDonald described certain aspects of her schizophrenic episode, especially during its acute onset, in a way quite reminiscent of a psychedelic experience.

> What I do want to explain, if I can, is the exaggerated state of awareness in which I lived before, during and after my acute illness. At first it was as if parts of my brain "awoke" which had been dormant, and I became interested in a wide assortment of people, events, places and ideas which normally would make no impression on me. Not knowing that I was ill, I made no attempt to understand what was happening. But there was some overwhelming significance in all this, produced either by God or Satan, and I felt that I was duty bound to ponder on each of these new interests, and the more I pondered the worse it became. The walk of a stranger on the street could be a "sign" to me which I must interpret. Every face in the windows of a passing streetcar would be engraved on my mind, all of them concentrating on me and trying to pass me some sort of message.

Ms. McDonald felt that her feelings while psychotic were much akin to the feelings of those who had ingested psychedelic drugs and reported "that I could talk to normal people who had the experience of taking mescaline or lysergic acid, and they would accept the things I told them about my adventures in mind without asking stupid questions."

An anonymous patient who had recovered from a catatonic schizophrenic episode reported that, during the initial phases of his decompensation, "It was also a time of inspiration and renewal . . . my capacities for esthetic appreciation and heightened sensory receptiveness, for vivid grasp of the qualities of living, and for an imaginative empathy were very keen at this time . . . I was particularly structuring the onset with the inspired nature of simple ordinary truths . . . love was also of great importance."

In an attempt to quantify psychedelic experiences and determine to what extent they were present in various groups of patients, Vincent Lamparella and I constructed an arbitrary scale based on typical psychedelic drug effects and then proceeded to rate the case histories of numerous psychiatric patients at the Johns Hopkins Hospital. It became evident that acute schizophrenic patients, especially in the early phases, reported a large number of events which were quite similar to those undergone by subjects ingesting psychedelic drugs. Such events were much rarer with chronic schizophrenics, except during an acute exacerbation of their illness.

Thus it seems as if something very much like psychedelic drug experiences are a frequent occurrence early in schizophrenic illness. Aldous Huxley, with his characteristic perspicacity, sensed this similarity, even though he himself had never been schizophrenic. At one point while under the influence of mescaline, he was entranced by his perceptions of a garden and then realized

it was inexpressibly wonderful, wonderful to the point, almost, of being terrifying. And suddenly I had an inkling of what it must feel like to be mad. Schizophrenia has its heavens as well as its hells and purgatories. I remember what an old friend, dead these many years, told me about his mad wife. One day in the early stages of the disease when she still had her lucid intervals, he had gone to talk to her about their children. She listened for a time, then cut him short. How could he bear to waste his time on a couple of absent children, when all that really mattered, here and now, was the unspeakable beauty of the patterns he made, in this brown tweed jacket, every time he moved his arms?

The British psychiatrist R. D. Laing also has emphasized how an acute schizophrenic decompensation can be a transcendental experience which he views as sometimes therapeutic. Schizophrenia for Laing is often a cleansing process in which old suppressed emotional wounds are brought to the surface and lived through whereupon they cease to trouble the patient, who is accordingly now "cured." As Laing puts it "madness need not be all breakdown. It may also be breakthrough. It is potentially liberation and renewal as well as enslavement and existential death."

Laing feels that the transcendental (we might call it psychedelic) features of the schizophrenic illness contain the kernel of cure. Only by allowing a patient to become grossly psychotic, in order that he might have such an experience, can he emerge from his illness in solid mental health, reintegrated into the everyday world, but retaining in the back of his mind the sense of potential oneness with the universe which is the mainspring of his healing.

As an example of a patient who underwent a schizophrenic break and its "natural" cure, he cites a patient of Karl Jaspers who described his gradual decomposition after which

> then came illumination . . . A larger and more comprehensive self emerged and I could abandon the previous personality with its entire entourage. I saw this earlier personality could never enter transcendental realms . . . A new life began for me and from now I felt different from other people. A self that consisted of conventional lies, shams, self-deceptions, memory images, a self just like that of other people, grew in me again but behind and above it stood a greater and more comprehensive self which impressed me with something of what is eternal, unchanging, immortal

and inviolable and which ever since that time has been my protector and refuge. I believe it would be good for many if they were acquainted with a higher self and that there are people who have attained this goal in fact by kinder means.

Laing thus feels that the mental health of most people is a rather tenuous business, and that in some ways the most sane people are those who have at one time or another themselves been insane. As he puts it,

True sanity entails in one way or another the disillusion of the normal ego, that false self competently adjusted to our alienated social reality; the emergence of the "inner" archetypal mediators of divine power; and through this death a rebirth, and the eventual reestablishment of a new kind of ego functioning, the ego now being the servant of the divine, no longer its betrayer.

4

What Is Schizophrenia?

Schizophrenia is a bad disease. Almost everything one can imagine that could be wrong is wrong in the mental life of the schizophrenic. His thinking processes are greatly impaired. He suffers from all sorts of delusions, which may be terrifying, or comforting, or both at the same time. He may be confused and unable to comprehend what is going on about him. On the other hand, he may be all too acutely aware of what people are saying and may know exactly what they mean, often far better than they know it themselves.

Yet even with this heightened comprehension, the schizophrenic patient has no solace; for he cannot assess the significance of the information appropriately, instead magnifying and distorting it out of all proportions. Often his discourse is halting, with long pauses which seem to stem from a sort of mental, and perhaps more fundamentally, emotional block.

The schizophrenic hears voices, eerie, unworldly sounds, or terrifying, threatening admonitions. He may see awesome visions. His emotional life is a real jungle. He is terrified of other people and will go to great lengths to retreat from them. In fact, many psychiatrists feel that it is this dread of other people, the "interpersonal terror," which is fundamental to schizophrenia and gives rise to the disorders of thinking and perceiving. The latter arises as a way of warding off the emotional threat of other people. By distorting thinking processes and altering perceptions, it might be possible to blunt the threat posed by other human beings.

But no one truly understands the fear of others or whatever else provides the nucleus for the tumultuous spectrum of symptoms harbored by most schizophrenic patients. Despite thousands of scientific publications and innumerable psychiatric theories, no one is yet certain as to what is fundamental to the schizophrenic process. Hallucinations, hearing or seeing what is not present in the environment, are the most dramatic of schizophrenic symptoms. Yet most psychiatrists hold that they are only secondary symptoms which arise as a means of dealing with more primary difficulties in thinking and feeling. That is what many psychiatrists think, but they don't really know. Psychoanalysts have brilliantly deciphered the psychological meaning of seemingly meaningless utterings, delusions and hallucinations of schizophrenics. They can understand and even relate them back to interactions of the patients with their parents in early years. But they have never been able to explain why this particular patient, out of the many thousands who must have had just as traumatic parental influences, was elected to join the ranks of those with schizophrenia, while the others escaped with neuroses or perhaps were fortunate enough to turn out "normal."

Insuperable though the task may seem, it is still important to make psychological sense out of the varied symptoms of schizophrenia. If one were to understand what is going on at a psychological level, perhaps this would suggest what might be transpiring in terms of the physiology and biochemistry of the brain. One might then have a clue as to the cardinal, fundamental biochemical abnormality, if one actually exists. Discerning with precision a biochemical fault which accounts for the symptoms of schizophrenia would probably rank as one of the greatest scientific achievements in human history. Moreover, with a little luck, the optimal therapy and perhaps even cure would then be only a matter of a few simple and obvious technological maneuvers.

Just what is schizophrenia? One medical dictionary says:

> Schizophrenic reaction is one of a group of psychotic reactions, often beginning after adolescence or in young adulthood, characterized by fundamental disturbances in reality relationships and concept formations, with associated affective, behavioral and intellectual disturbances in varying degrees and mixtures. These reactions are marked by a tendency to withdraw from reality, inappropriate moods, unpredictable disturbances in stream of thought, regressive tendencies to the point of deterioration, and often hallucinations and delusions.

While such a definition hardly solves any of our problems, it at least poses them clearly enough. For it describes the many manifestations of schizophrenia, invading all aspects of reality relationships. One important point which it fails to emphasize is that the disturbance which the schizophrenic experiences in his encounters with reality occurs in a setting of fairly clear consciousness. The patient is oriented to person, place, and time, which simply means that he knows who he is, where he is, and the date (although it may not be easy to drag from him all this information). These features distinguish a schizophrenic psychosis from an organic psychosis, such as one that occurs with a high fever or after ingesting a toxic drug. In an organic psychosis, the patient is usually disoriented and very confused, and one can usually pinpoint the source of the trouble, whether it be advanced syphilis, arteriosclerosis, or some noxious drug. On the other hand, in the "functional" psychoses, of which schizophrenia is the best example, no such causes are apparent, and the patient fails to manifest any of the typical "organic" traits.

With so many different manifestations, why do people insist on considering schizophrenia as a single disease? Is there any evidence one way or the other? Where did the whole idea begin?

A Brief History

Nineteenth-century European medicine was dominated by the pathologists, specialists who delineated illnesses by examining under the microscope diseased organs of the body and then relating the abnormalities they described to the patients' symptoms. They were highly successful in applying the scientific method to medical practice. Clinical disease entities could be described meaningfully by relating them to the pathology. It turned out that patients whose diseased organs had a uniformly characteristic appearance under the microscope often had closely similar symptoms.

Psychiatry in the nineteenth century was greatly influenced by the success of the pathologists.

There was a flurry of enthusiasm that the major mental illnesses could be solved, because of the enormously successful demonstration that "general paralysis of the insane," a condition with psychiatric symptoms as well as a loss if intellectual capacity, was simply an advanced form of syphilis. Such patients may ultimately become paralyzed, but their most dramatic manifestations are emotional. They often become elatedly grandiose and somewhat confused. The philosopher Friedrich Nietzsche succumbed to syphilis of the brain, and I suspect that this illness contributed to some of the extravagance of his later works. By the turn of the century, clinical suspicion became certainty when the syphilitis organism or "spirochete" was directly demonstrated in the brains of these patients.

The German physician Kahlbaum divined part of the package of schizophrenia when he realized that a specific assortment of symptoms fitted a large group of patients quite nicely, patients who went through a series of successive stages with a bad outcome. This was catatonia. His catatonic patients began by being melancholic (somewhat depressed) and then entered a stage of what he referred to as "mania," which we would call "catatonic excitement," followed by a stupor leading gradually into more and more confusion and finally a mental deterioration. Unfortunately, as more patients accumulated who seemed to fit the major symptoms of catatonia, especially the excitement and stupor, it became clear that the typical course that Kahlbaum described was the exception rather than the rule. However, some features of catatonia did seem to apply to a reasonably sizable group of patients, and it was generally felt that this represented one of the first clear delineations of a psychotic disease process.

Spurred on by Kahlbaum's success, another German psychiatrist, Hecker, went on to describe a collection of symptoms called "hebephrenia," in which fairly young patients, usually in their teens, presented with a giggling form of psychosis with much more deterioration than occurred in catatonia.

Emil Kraepelin, a giant of nineteenth-century German psychiatry, adopted a productive approach. Since the anatomy of the brain had failed to provide a key to the nature of the various types of mental patients, he chose clinical outcome as his principal tool in making diagnoses. In this way, simply by making a diagnosis the psychiatrist would be in a position to predict the clinical course and eventual outcome.

Kraepelin separated patients who gradually deteriorated, mentally and emotionally, from those who tended to hold together and often recover. In so doing he ended up with two major entities which had a rather nice "fit". Patients with manic-depressive psychosis generally recovered from a given manic or depressive episode, enough so that they could often be discharged from the hospital though they might later suffer recurrence. In terms of their symptoms, manic-depressive patients seemed very much alike, and thus formed a neat diagnostic grouping.

By contrast, the other group was composed of a varied assortment including catatonia and hebephrenia, which Kraepelin labeled *dementia praecox*, meaning "mental deterioration of the young." These patients hallucinated, experienced delusions, disorders of emotional behavior, obstinate and negativistic behavior, and became progressively deteriorated. Despite such a disorganized mental life, they were generally quite alert and were clearly orientated to person, place and time. Among the subtypes included under the rubric of *dementia praecox* were the following: Hebephrenic patients were ones who tended to act inappropriately "silly" and deteriorate rapidly; catatonic patients would be either wildly excited and agitated or at other times totally immobile in a "catatonic stupor"; paranoid patients had prominent delusions of persecution or grandiosity. It has always seemed to me that Kraepelin was operating with few facts in hand and playing a guessing game. But his guesses were astute, for modern psychiatrists still regard his groupings as valid and have simply interchanged the word "schizophrenia" for *dementia praecox.*

There were a number of flaws in Kraepelin's reasoning. First, of course, is the fact that "dementia" is by no means the rule. Nowadays it is quite rare to find a schizophrenic who has deteriorated to the point of loss of his intellectual capacities. It is quite likely that Kraepelin and his predecessors flung about the term "dementia" far too loosely. What they saw as intellectual deterioration was more a result of being locked up in insane asylums for many years with little human contact than an effect of the mental illness itself. Modern treatment with drugs or exploratory psychotherapy or simply intense affection and attention by people who care has almost eliminated the form of deterioration which Kraepelin thought to be the hallmark of *dementia praecox.*

Another difficulty with Kraepelin's way of viewing the illness was simply that it does not really occur exclusively in young people. Paranoid schizophrenia, for instance, tends to make its appearance later on in the thirty to fifty age group.

Perhaps the greatest difficulty with Kraepelin's position is that he failed to clarify just what is crazy about these crazy people. He knew they were psychotic. He described many of their behaviors. However, he was reluctant to penetrate the "black box" of their mental functioning. In this way Kraepelin and all the other psychiatrists of his time were quite modern "behaviorists." B. F. Skinner would probably have admired their forbearance, since, as modern behaviorist dogma states, what goes on inside the head cannot be observed and therefore is not "science." Kraepelin was applying the rigors of the scientific method, borrowed from his colleagues in medicine and pathology, to clinical manifestations of behavior, long before the Skinnerians applied the "scientific method" to an experimental analysis of behavior.

But Kraepelin's approach did work. By pigeonholing certain patients in the class *dementia praecox*, he separated them from those afflicted with a purely organic form of brain deterioration. As another spinoff from his description of *dementia praecox*, Kraepelin threw into bold relief the condition of manic-depressive psychosis. For it soon became apparent that almost all hospitalized psychiatric patients either suffered from dementia praecox or possessed manic-depressive illness. And the latter turned out to be a clearly definable disease, reflecting a fairly homogeneous group of patients with a distinctive collection of symptoms and clinical course.

The next giant step forward was taken by the Swiss psychiatrist Eugen Bleuler, to whom we owe the designation "schizophrenia." Bleuler recognized an important and subtle point which Kraepelin, and many, many other psychiatrists, failed to appreciate. The universe of the severely mentally ill was not identical with the inhabitants of Kraepelin's hospital. There might be many patients who never required hospitalization but who still manifested the symptoms of *dementia praecox*. Bleuler did look outside the hospital and found patients whose symptoms would qualify them for the diagnosis of *dementia praecox* but who never deteriorated as they should have, according to Kraepelin. Moreover, there were other patients within the mental hospitals with *dementia praecox* who failed to deteriorate. Thus, Bleuler widened the net of potential candidates for *dementia praecox*, and at the same time injected a note of optimism by arguing that these patients need not all suffer an unhappy fate.

Bleuler's other major contribution was in trying to make some sense out of the mélange of his patients' symptoms. He rejected the cautious descriptive approach of nineteenth-century German psychiatry and ushered in the era of twentieth-century speculative, philosophic psychiatry which was to be carried to its ultimate by Sigmund Freud and the various schools of psychoanalysis. Bleuler speculated that the primary disorder in all patients with schizophrenia was a deficiency in the ability to form mental associative links. Patients did not think or feel in an orderly, logical way, and consequently the basic functions of their personality were divorced or split from each other. Many people tend to think that schizophrenia means "split personality" in the sense of multiple personalities as, for example, in the famous patient whose life story was told in the movie, *The Three Faces of Eve.* The schizophrenic should only be so lucky. He cannot integrate a single personality, much less pull off with histrionic verve an effective presentation of three of them.

Bleuler's notion that the primary symptoms of

schizophrenia lay in faulty mental associations was a theoretical construct, existing more in the mind of Bleuler than in the behavior of schizophrenic patients. For something which is more directly observable, Bleuler described how the proposed primary disturbance in mental associations could then lead to a number of secondary symptoms. For instance, the disturbance in mental associations might well be expected to result in blocking of thoughts and feelings. Most of us have experienced mental blockages on occasion when we were quite anxious. We begin a sentence, knowing full well what we mean to say, but then freeze in the middle of it and cannot regain our train of thought. This sort of disturbance constantly invades the thinking processes of the schizophrenic patient. Other secondary symptoms are a withdrawal of feeling and thought from reality, resulting in extremely self-centered "autistic" behavior. Moreover, as a consequence of the disturbed associations, schizophrenics are profoundly ambivalent in their feelings about almost everyone and everything. This would hardly be surprising, since a splitting, or lack of integration, of associations might readily result in the existence side by side of elation and depression, love and hate.

As for basic ideas about what the entity "schizophrenia" involves, there has not been much advance since the days of Bleuler. Adolf Meyer, the Swiss psychiatrist who emigrated to the United States and became the father of American psychiatry, devoted much attention to the subject. He agreed with all that Bleuler had enunciated but went on to stress ways in which these changes might come about in individual patients. He urged psychiatrists to study their patients from the beginning of life in order to trace the gradual deterioration of their way of living. He speculated that "faulty habits" such as brooding or too much fantasy might gradually be transformed into schizophrenic symptoms. Thus, Meyer was the first eminent psychiatrist to espouse the viewpoint that schizophrenia might stem from environmental influences rather than brain biochemistry. The disease might simply be a product of the wrong sort of mother, father, school experiences, and so on. This way of thinking is in marked contrast to Bleuler. Even though Bleuler divined at length about the feelings and mental goings on of the schizophrenic patient, he always adhered to the belief that the disease had some organic basis. Though the pathology had not been revealed by microscopic examination of the brain, perhaps some day chemical studies would reveal the toxin at fault.

Sigmund Freud hardly ever saw a schizophrenic patient. It is a remarkable and little appreciated circumstance that the father of so much of twentieth-century psychiatry, a man who issued numerous pronouncements on the nature of schizophrenia, directly dealt with fewer schizophrenics than do some modern-day medical students. The reason seems straightforward and very sad. The hierarchy of Austrian university psychiatric hospitals was quite anti-Semitic at the time, so that Freud was forced to confine himself to work with office patients, who were generally only neurotic.

His major contribution to the study of schizophrenia lies in his essay interpreting the memoirs of Judge Daniel Paul Schreber, a sophisticated paranoid schizophrenic. Freud devoted much of the essay to an analysis of how paranoid thinking was a way of dealing with unacceptable homosexual impulses. Thus the wish "I love the man" is denied and transformed to "I hate him," which the patient then projects onto the outside world with the resultant paranoid delusion "He hates me." Freud also focused on the way in which the schizophrenic individual withdraws his emotions from concerns· about other people into a total absorption with himself. For Freud, the delusions and hallucinations were not the essence of madness but manifestations of residual mental health, distorted ways whereby the patient strives desperately to reestablish contact with the outside world.

From this brief historical survey, probably the only thing which is quite clear is the great ignorance of the psychiatric community as to the fundamental nature of the schizophrenic disturbance, an ignorance which has not changed much in the past hundred years. Certain crucial questions have failed to yield to the plethora of investigations of schizophrenia. For instance, is schizophrenia one disease or a group of diseases? Eugen Bleuler always hedged his bets. Even though he postulated a common fundamental disorder, he still always referred to "the group of schizophrenias."

Capitalizing on this confused situation, Thomas Szasz has made himself the maverick of American psychiatry by debunking all the standard psychiatric categories. As for schizophrenia he concludes, "The problem of schizophrenia, which many consider to be the core problem of psychiatry today, may be truly akin to the 'problem of the ether. . . .' To put it simply: there is no such problem."

Is Schizophrenia Inherited?

Thus we are not absolutely certain if schizophrenia as a discrete entity exists at all. If we accept, as I do, that there is a real disease or diseases called schizophrenia,

another knotty question must be posed. Is schizophrenia psychogenic, the result of a wicked schizo-
phrénia-provoking or "schizophrenogenic" mother? Or
is some concrete breakdown in the brain responsible
for the illness?

A partial answer has come from a variety of genetic
studies of schizophrenia. The rationale is simple. Let us
assume that schizophrenia is an inherited disease determined by genetic factors. One simply sees if schizophrenia "runs" in families. If it does, one then determines the pattern of inheritance. What percentage of
the children of schizophrenics develop the disease
themselves? Must the disease be present in both the
mother's and the father's families for a child to suffer a
breakdown?

Many family studies have been performed over the
years. Schizophrenia certainly occurs more frequently
in the families of schizophrenics than in nonschizophrenic families. However, one can readily argue
that this is quite consistent with a psychogenic rather
than a genetic basis for the disease. For a disturbed
parent who is "schizophrenogenic" will be exerting
influences upon all the children so that if one becomes
schizophrenic it is quite likely that others will as well.

The question of parental influences on a patient's
siblings can be overcome by comparing identical and
fraternal twins. Identical twins develop from the same
egg, hence share identical genetic make-ups. Fraternal
twins emerge from fertilization of two different eggs and
so are no more similar genetically than any two siblings.
Identical twins are exposed to the same home environment, but fraternal twins are as well. Accordingly, if the
ministrations of an intolerable mother are responsible
for the disease and she drives one twin crazy, the other

twin should have the same chance of succumbing whether he is identical or fraternal.

The eminent student of human genetics Franz Kallmann found that if one identical twin became schizophrenic, his co-twin had an eighty-five percent chance of becoming schizophrenic. On the other hand, if a fraternal twin was schizophrenic, his co-twin had only a fifteen percent chance of developing the disease. This fifteen percent "concordance rate" turns out to be the same as the concordance rate for siblings who are not twins.

There have been many other twin studies since Kallmann's work. Though many of them have failed to obtain as dramatic differences between the concordance rate for schizophrenia in identical and fraternal twins, almost all have come up with the same trend as Kallmann. Such findings would argue strongly that schizophrenia is an inherited disease. Some biological, presumably biochemical deficiency is genetically determined. Thus there may truly exist a "toxin" or missing chemical in schizophrenia awaiting discovery by some fortunate investigator.

The experiments with twins provide fairly convincing evidence that a strong genetic element determines whether someone will become schizophrenic. At this point it is very easy to fall into the trap of asserting that schizophrenia is a "genetic disease." But stating cautiously that there is a "genetic component" in determining the occurrence of schizophrenia is a far cry from claiming that the disease is caused only by bad genes. Let it be granted that if one twin is schizophrenic, his identical twin is very likely also to become schizophrenic sooner or later, and, therefore, these two unfortunates must have inherited some genetic factor predisposing toward schizophrenia. At the same time we must not forget that there might well be many other parents, not themselves schizophrenics, but carrying the "bad genes" which they might even transmit to their children; yet the children remain normal. We don't know how many such parents and children exist, but there may be many of them. In those cases, one would argue that the schizophrenic genes were not enough to trigger the disease. Rather, some environmental stress was necessary to set it off.

Very recently several investigators, particularly Seymour Kety, David Rosenthal, Paul Wender, and Leonard Heston of the United States as well as Fini Schulsinger in Denmark, have been able to increase greatly the sophistication of the genetic studies of schizophrenia and have turned up several illuminating facts about the disease.

Most of the work of Kety, Rosenthal, Wender, and Schulsinger was conducted in Denmark, a country in which one can keep track via the *folkeregister*, a population tabulation of the life history and whereabouts from birth to death of almost every human being in Denmark. In this way they could track down the location of all the relatives of people who had been in mental hospitals as long as twenty or more years ago.

In one study, they selected from the list of all children adopted in Denmark over a twenty-three-year span those who subsequently became schizophrenic. They then examined the frequency of mental illness in both the biologic and the adoptive parents of these patients. For a control comparison group they took adopted children who never became mentally ill and scrutinized their biological and adoptive parents for mental illness. Since most of the children were adopted less than one month after birth, they grew up without ever seeing or knowing their biological parents. Because of this it is unlikely that the biological mother would have had any chance to "teach" her child how to be schizophrenic.

What might one expect from such a study? If schizophrenia is caused by stifling influences of schizophrenogenic parents, one would anticipate that it was the adoptive parents who were responsible for schizophrenia in the children and who accordingly would manifest some sort of bizarre behavioral traits. On the other hand, if schizophrenia is determined primarily by genetic factors, one would anticipate quite a bit of psychopathology in the biological parents, probably with a substantial chunk of schizophrenia and related disorders. As it turned out, schizophrenia and related disorders occurred much more frequently in the biological parents and families than in the adoptive families. In fact, the adopted parents and families of the schizophrenic children had little more likelihood of having mental disturbance than the biological or adoptive parents of nonschizophrenic adoptees. Clearly something genetic was going on.

Besides confirming what we suspected all along from the twin studies, this investigation gave extra dividends. Earlier we raised the question of whether there were different types of schizophrenia. One fairly solid way of distinguishing subtypes of schizophrenia would be to see if some run in families while others are not inherited. Accordingly, Seymour Kety divided his schizophrenic adoptees into three groups according to their symptoms. Some were diagnosed as having chronic schizophrenia, because their illness had developed quite insidiously over many years, while others were called "acute schizophrenics," because they had appeared fairly well adjusted until they deteriorated abruptly in relationship to some stressful event. The acute schizophrenics tended to recover fairly rapidly, while the chronic schizophrenics went downhill over the years. A third category were patients diagnosed as borderline schizophrenics. These individuals did not quite fulfill all the diagnostic criteria for schizophrenia. Yet, even though they could communicate reasonably clearly and appear poised in interviews, their thinking was a bit vague, they had experienced episodes of feeling strange and confused under stress when they would have something akin to a "micropsychosis," and they were never happy.

As expected, the patients with chronic schizophrenia had a very high incidence of schizophrenia-related disorders in their biological families. On the other hand, for the acute schizophrenics there were no cases of schizophrenia or anything resembling it in their biological relatives. Surprisingly, for the borderline schizophrenics, who seemed closest to normal in their everyday functioning, the likelihood of schizophrenia in their biological families was just as high as for the chronic schizophrenics.

All of this suggests that acute schizophrenia is a completely different disease from chronic or borderline schizophrenia. Acute schizophrenia does not seem to run in families. Perhaps it is some sort of reaction to extreme stress, which could conceivably afflict almost anyone exposed to an overwhelmingly traumatic situation. For example, it is well known that many soldiers, otherwise normal, become psychotic in the battlefield, but recover rapidly when removed from the battlefront and do not become mentally ill thereafter.

One wonders what the borderline schizophrenics have in common with the chronic schizophrenics. They do resemble each other in that their disturbance has often been a life-long affair. Borderline schizophrenics are people who have never been quite crazy but at the same time have never been able to function normally in society. They gravitate to life styles in which idiosyncratic ways of thinking and feeling are accepted, such as bohemian, "hippie" cultures.

Dr. Leonard Heston at the University of Iowa unearthed perhaps even more provocative notions about schizophrenia. He evaluated adopted children born to schizophrenic mothers and compared their fate to that of adopted children born to mothers with no known history of psychiatric disorder. In all cases, the children were separated from their mothers within two weeks of birth. Seventeen percent of the children of schizophrenic mothers became clearly schizophrenic, while none of the children of nonschizophrenic mothers became schizophrenic. Again, Heston reaffirms the importance of genetic inheritance in the development of schizophrenia. Even more interestingly, he found that about half of all the children of schizophrenic mothers developed some very major psychosocial disability. About twenty percent of them developed life-long "sociopathic" behavior. Thus these individuals lived a life distinguished by antisocial behavior of an impulsive, illogical nature. They were arrested many times for assault, battery, or poorly planned impulsive thefts. Some were homosexual, others alcoholics, and a few were narcotic addicts. This would suggest that the genes transmitting schizophrenia might often be expressed in sociopathic behavior. Accordingly, the biological disease schizophrenia may account for a much wider spectrum of people with abnormal behavior than simply those who fit a strict diagnosis of schizophrenia.

Heston unearthed yet other surprising and tantalizing data. For instance, almost twenty percent of the children of schizophrenic mothers, but no children of nonschizophrenic mothers, had very striking musical ability and about fifteen percent had unusually strong religious feelings. It is easy to reconcile the high incidence of religiosity as a means of coming to grips with emotional problems, but what of the musical talent? This raises specters of the widely held but presumed mythical notion that creative artistic and musical abilities go hand and hand with mental illness.

Other, nongenetic sorts of experiments also suggest that schizophrenia is not caused by the emotional influence of the child's parents over many years but is related to something which either occurred at birth, occurred before birth, or was genetic. Dr. William Pollin at the National Institute of Mental Health in Bethesda, Maryland, compared a number of characteristics of 100 pairs of identical twins in which only one of the twins was schizophrenic. He evaluated many measures ranging from how they behaved in childhood to their physical health. Not surprisingly, the feature that best differentiated the two groups was whether or not they were neurotic as children. The schizophrenic co-twin was sixteen times as likely to have been severely neurotic as a child than was his sibling. He was also much more likely to be submissive, sensitive, a serious worrier, obedient, dependent, quiet, and shy.

Of course, none of this is surprising, and it does not offer much in the way of deciding whether it was the home environment or some more biological factor which was responsible for the schizophrenic illness. If the schizophrenia had been produced by some noxious emotional bearhug of the mother, one would expect to see the consequences of her activities on the behavior of the twin elected to become schizophrenic many years before his deterioration. And, of course, if a biological factor such as genetic influences or prenatal disturbances had given rise to the schizophrenic influence we would also anticipate some behavioral aberrations at an early age.

What is most striking were physical differences Pollin detected between the twins at an early age. These were apparent even at birth. The twin who became schizophrenic was considerably more likely to have been the lighter of the two children at birth. In twelve out of fifteen pairs of twins, the schizophrenic twin was lighter at birth. The schizophrenic twin was also four times as likely as his sibling to have experienced some complications at birth, particularly difficulty with breathing. Throughout childhood, the future schizophrenic also differed from his sibling. He tended to be weaker, shorter, and slower in learning to walk. Moreover, he was much more likely to have suffered some sort of central nervous system illness as a child, such as meningitis.

By contrast the twin who failed to develop schizophrenia was quite frequently the more intelligent one in I.Q. tests. He did better at school and was generally the spokesman for the pair of twins. He was much more likely to be outgoing and lively, to be a leader among his peers, and to be athletic.

Clearly the future schizophrenic is less favored constitutionally to deal with the world than his twin. He is certainly more vulnerable, more dependent, and a weaker person. Presumably, this would have implications for his self-image and identity in the world. He would be less able to deal with the stress of everyday life and might well succumb to psychic disintegration. Instead of emphasizing the emotional weakness which results from physical weakness at birth, one might just as well emphasize apparent brain damage which seems to predominate in the future schizophrenic co-twin.

Of course at this point we must start wondering whether or not there is any difference between talking about the patient's "psychological" versus his "neurological" vulnerability. One thing, however, is clear. These were identical twins. They had the same genetic endowment. Yet one became schizophrenic and not the other, so it is not the genes alone which make a person schizophrenic. Environmental influences are of great importance in transforming what is a genetic potentiality into manifest schizophrenic illness. Subtle differences in a person's ability to deal with the world physically, such as his motor coordination and muscle strength, as well as his ability to deal with the world emotionally and intellectually, make a big difference in determining the final outcome.

5

Schizophrenic Thinking and Feeling

Granted that the tendency to become schizophrenic is an inherited trait. Moreover, it is quite likely that whatever is inherited is common to a number of different forms of schizophrenia and may even be present in some people with nonschizophrenic disturbances. Thus, from genetic studies, we develop new confidence that schizophrenia does represent a discrete disease or cluster of diseases. Still, we have yet to solve the question posed at the beginning of the book. What are the cardinal features of schizophrenia? Was Eugen Bleuler right? Is there some key abnormality in mental or emotional function which gives rise to all the other symptoms? Suppose we can't pin down such a fundamental abnormality. Is it still possible to think about schizophrenia in a way that will help us relate it to what is already known and what may be revealed in the future about brain physiology and chemistry in order to help find a metabolic abnormality which is the expression of the "schizophrenic gene"?

To do this, let us first describe the major clinical features of most schizophrenic patients. Since schizophrenic disturbances in thinking and feeling probably make up the "essence" of the disease, they should come first. And since the views of Eugen Bleuler have not been much improved upon in sixty years, let us initially examine his notions.

Bleuler was fascinated by the then recent writings of Sigmund Freud, which he learned about through his colleague, Carl Jung, an intense disciple of Freud's. Because psychoanalysis is especially concerned with the interior of patients' psyches, Bleuler was eager to explore what went on inside the minds of patients with dementia praecox. He clung to the Kraepelin's doctrine that all of these patients had something in common, despite their great disparity in overt symptoms, although he did always retain in his writings the caveat that this condition may well represent a group of diseases rather than a single entity. In his classis monograph, *Dementia Praecox, or, The Group of Schizophrenias*, which virtually everyone in the psychiatric profession will agree represents the most important book ever written about this disease, he felt that he had discovered the common denominator.

Because it is just such a common denominator, or primary deficit in mental functioning, which we would like to uncover, let us examine Bleuler's reasoning in considerable detail. And since the modern clinical definition of schizophrenia continues to be almost identical to the original Bleulerian formulation, we can restrict our description of clinical schizophrenia largely to Bleuler's rich and lucid writing. In this way we may best avoid the gross distortions and confusions which have arisen in the sixty years since Bleuler published his monograph. During this time textbook after textbook has always developed the notion of schizophrenia almost exactly according to Bleuler—but generally Bleuler taken from secondary sources, since for some bizarre reason Bleuler's classic monograph, published in German in 1911, was not translated into English or any other language until 1950.

Right at the outset of his book Bleuler lets us in on the punchline, telling us just what he thinks is wrong with schizophrenics by renaming the disease. He calls it "schizophrenia, because (as I hope to demonstrate) the splitting of the different psychic functions is one of its most important characteristics. For the sake of convenience, I use the word in the singular although it is apparent that the group includes several diseases (an important reservation, which too many psychiatrists have overlooked)."

Bleuler felt that the disease was characterized by "a specific type of alteration of thinking, feeling, and relation to the external world which appears nowhere else in this particular fashion." He understood quite clearly the difference between schizophrenia and organic disorders of mental function and emphasized that schizophrenia differs from these because, in schizophrenia "primary disturbances of perception, orientation, or memory are not demonstrable."

He coined the word "schizophrenia" from two Greek words which together mean "a splitting of the mind." What he meant by "mind" is both the intellectual and the emotional mind, so that for him the defects were "mental associations" and "affect" (which means feeling state). Thus, according to Bleuler, what is fundamentally disturbed in a schizophrenic patient is his ability to integrate his thoughts and feelings into a coherent meshwork so that thinking may be meaningful and feelings and actions may be sensibly goal-oriented. Of these two psychic functions, Bleuler and all subsequent psychiatrists have laid the greatest emphasis on the disturbance in mental associations which results in what is commonly referred to as a "formal thought disorder," the *sine qua non* for the diagnosis of schizophrenia. To reemphasize what Bleuler meant by a schizophrenic thought disorder, it is worthwhile to quote him directly: "In the normal thinking process, the numerous actual and latent images combine to determine each association." Here Bleuler is trying to convey the notion that most normal thinking, even of quite simple concepts, involves a tying together of numerous threads of ideas or mental images both conscious or unconscious. His emphasis on the role of unconscious processes here reminds us of his fascination at that time with the then recent publications of Freud.

> In schizophrenia, however, single images or whole combinations may be rendered ineffective, in an apparent haphazard fashion. Instead, thinking operates with ideas and concepts which have no, or a completely insufficient, connection with the main idea and should therefore be excluded from the thought process. The result is that thinking becomes confused, bizarre, incorrect, abrupt. Sometimes, all the associative threads fail and the thought chain is totally interrupted; after such "blocking," ideas may emerge which have no recognizable connection with preceding ones.

Many people have interpreted Bleuler to mean that the mental associations of schizophrenics are "loose" and that such looseness in thinking is uniquely schizophrenic. But this is not really correct. One must be quite specific in describing and applying the notion of disturbance in mental associations to schizophrenics. For instance, an individual in a manic state speaks with "loose associations." Witness the following utterances by a typically manic patient, "Things are great. Let me buy you dinner. I think I'll buy the restaurant. Food is all that matters; I can't have enough. Food is for the fit. I feel fantastic, fabulous. You are fabulous, gorgeous, beautiful." What is wrong with this manic patient is simply that he is thinking and speaking so quickly that there is no time to screen ideas for their logical relevance to his main thought before they spew forth from his mouth. Although the associations are "loose" they do have a logical link with the main theme. Schizophrenics tie their ideas together in a much crazier way.

Proverbs Parallel Schizophrenia—Or Do They?

Many people have tried to delimit and quantify the presumed defect in schizophrenic thinking. One technique which has gained great favor in clinical psychiatry is proverb interpretation. Its popularity stems from the fact that it can be readily utilized during initial interviews with patients. As long ago as 1931 several investigators had reported abnormalities in the way schizophrenics interpreted proverbs. Dr. John Benjamin in the late 1930s experimented with a set of proverbs which have now become classic tools in examining patients suspected of schizophrenia. For instance when one patient was asked to interpret the proverb "When the cat's away, the mice will play," he answered, "When there is nobody watching they do things they wouldn't if the cat were there." Another patient responded, "If there isn't any cat around, the mice will monkey around and maybe get into things." When asked to explain the meaning of "A rolling stone gathers no moss," one patient responded, "A stone that keeps rolling doesn't stay still long enough to have moss grow on it."

Clearly what is wrong is that these patients are interpreting proverbs literally, concretely. Many psychiatrists, upon hearing such interpretations, leap to the diagnosis of schizophrenia. Unfortunately they fail to recognize what Dr. Benjamin discovered in the 1930s and what had been known even decades before Benjamin's work, namely, that individuals with organic mental disturbance or even mild mental deficiency will interpret proverbs just as concretely. The only types of proverb interpretation which Dr. Benjamin found to be unmistakably schizophrenic were those which are bizarre and related primarily to the private fantasy world of the patient. Sometimes this private thinking of the schizophrenic seems on first glance to be profound. Thus one patient interpreted "A rolling stone gathers no moss" as "That a person who is always busy doesn't stop for reflection, doesn't grow in mental and moral stature." Perhaps we could find in such utterances a clue as to why throughout history fairly well-organized schizophrenics have been able to gather about them flocks of disciples who have elevated their delusional statements to the rank of prophecy and philosophy.

Sorting Things Out

In any event, insofar as a literal interpretation of proverbs is shared by patients with organic brain damage, it is unlikely that the literalness of the schizophrenic is a key to his peculiar disturbance in mental functioning. Many other studies of the "concrete" intellectual behavior of the schizophrenic patient suffer from the same criticism. For instance, Kurt Goldstein and Martin Scheerer developed a sorting test patterned after similar sorting tests which were pioneered by the famous Russian psychologist Vigotsky. In these tests objects are to be sorted into classes, which can be established on the basis of similar colors or similar shapes. Someone who is presumably normal and can think abstractly will group blocks of varying shades of a given color together. Goldstein found that schizophrenics could not abstract such concepts as efficiently as normals and tended to sort objects on very concrete grounds, requiring for instance that the "blue" category be limited only to blocks with identical shades of blue.

Goldstein even went on to theorize as to how such concrete thinking might explain the other symptoms of schizophrenics. If one behaves concretely rather than abstractly, one's life will be "governed to an abnormal degree by outer world stimuli which present themselves and by images, ideas, and thought which act upon him at the moment." This would occur because the schizophrenic patient would be unable to abstract what is important from what is not important and hence would have to pay attention to everything. If he pays attention to everything, then the world will be "too much to deal with," and it would be easy to imagine how he might retreat from such an overwhelming onslaught of stimuli to an inner world of fantasy.

The one insuperable difficulty with such a theory is that, as Goldstein himself had observed, patients with organic brain lesions (in this case World War I veterans with bullet wounds in the head) display just as concrete an attitude in Goldstein's sorting tests as the schizophrenics but never develop any of the other stigmata of schizophrenic illness.

Many other people have described the thinking of schizophrenics in similar ways. Some describe how the reasoning of schizophrenics fails to obey the laws of Aristotelian logic. Others point out how such difficulties in reasoning resemble very much the thinking processes of small children or of primitive peoples. All of these workers seem to be pointing to the same sorts of thinking abnormalities which, unfortunately, are just as characteristic of people with mental deficiency or other organic brain damage as of a schizophrenia.

Fright Makes for Crazy Thoughts

Harry Stack Sullivan, the eminent American psychiatrist, was active in the late 1930s when it was popular to look on schizophrenic thinking as concrete, literal, or paralogical. He noticed in the language of his schizophrenic patients the same strange patterns of reasoning as had the other psychiatrists, but he chose to explain them rather differently. He emphasized that most people use language in order to get something they want, to derive satisfaction. The schizophrenic, on the other hand, has known for a long time that he will never be satisfied, can never have what he wants, has no hope of truly communicating his feelings to others. Moreover, the world is for him a frightening, very dangerous place. He must use every tool at his disposal to develop some sort of feeling of security. Since he does not view language as particularly useful for communicating, he uses it instead to attain a feeling of personal security.

The schizophrenic patient tends to overgeneralize the true significance of threats. When given a traffic ticket, he feels he has been labeled a murderer. If Mother shouts at him, he fears she will kill him. The simplest way to nullify such threats or at least blunt their impact is to deny their general significance and focus only on the most limited, nonthreatening, and concrete aspects of each event. Hence, in contrast to the other theorizers, Harry Stack Sullivan seems to have felt that schizophrenics generalized and abstracted much more, albeit in a distorted way, than did normal individuals. Any apparently concrete behavior is simply a defense against the threat posed by a reality in which every happening perceived is generalized to an extent that it poses horrors of an enormity which can scarcely be imagined.

Feelings

Thus Harry Stack Sullivan felt that disorders of schizophrenic thought followed from their terror of the world. His ideas suggest that we would do well to take close heed to what Bleuler considered to be the second "primary disturbance" in schizophrenics, a disorder of feeling or "affectivity." Chronic schizophrenics don't even seem to show feelings at all. Their faces are emotionless. Psychiatrists classically refer to this state as a "blunting of affect." Bleuler assumed that it was this loss of feeling which was responsible for the apparent indifference of many patients to their ultimate fate. He described many pathetic examples in which

the sense of self-preservation is often reduced to zero. The patients do not bother anymore about whether they starve or not, whether they lie on a snow bank or on a red hot oven.

During a fire in a hospital a number of patients had to be led
out of the threatened wards; they themselves would never
have moved from their places; they would have allowed
themselves to be suffocated or burnt without showing any
affective response. Illnesses, threats of every possible evil
will not disturb the peace [of many a schizophrenic].

(Bleuler must have had a rather morbid sense of humor,
experienced some lack of insight, or simply been writing hastily to suggest that a schizophrenic is really ever
experiencing any "peace.") What happens to others is
of course no concern to them. One patient killed another; his wardmates do not find it necessary to call the
attendant. A student almost choked the life out of his
mother; he cannot understand why such a fuss is made
over "a few harsh words! . . . Schizophrenics can write
whole autobiographies without manifesting the least bit
of emotion. They will describe their suffering and their
actions as if it were a theme in physics."

Many modern existentialist psychiatrists, as we shall
see later, would greatly doubt whether schizophrenics,
even when "burnt out," are truly deficient in emotionali-
ty. Instead, they would maintain that these patients are
so weighed down by overriding and intolerable emotions that to stay alive they must hide their feelings from
the world and, as far as is possible, from themselves.
Bleuler himself realized this to a certain degree, since
he could in fact directly witness such hyperemotionality
in early patients and indeed commented, "At the beginning of the disease we often see an oversensitivity, so
that the patients consciously and deliberately isolate
themselves in order to avoid everything that might
arouse affect, even though they may still have some
interest in life. Latent schizophrenics may appear almost too labile in their affect, almost sanguine." Bleuler

emphasized that whether a given patient was displaying too much, too little, or just the right quantity of affect, there was something abnormal about its qualitative nature. In some patients large amounts of feeling may be forthcoming, but it is all seemingly lacking in depth. Others will display lively feeling in certain directions, but respond like blank walls to other situations.

What is more primary, the disorder in thinking, or the abnormality of feelings? Much of the twentieth-century psychiatry has been dominated at least in the United States, by psychoanalytic influences. The great contribution of psychoanalysis is its focus upon developing in its practitioners an expertise at dredging up people's feelings. Accordingly, there has been a great interest in the abnormality of feeling states in schizophrenic individuals.

One psychoanalyst, Sandor Rado, has formulated a complete theory of schizophrenia based on the difficulty schizophrenics have in experiencing pleasure, which he calls "anhedonia." The idea is simple. A schizophrenic, for one reason or another, since earliest childhood, has never been able to experience happiness. Nothing has ever been enjoyable for him. Viewing the world as a lackluster place where all people and experiences are similarly bland and devoid of vital interest, he soon has no motivation to encounter his environment. A retreat from the world to an inner life of fantasy in which infantile wishes can be gratified is much more fun. Since this private mental life has no need of symbols and language shared by other people, it is not surprising that bizarre, illogical, and "loose" thinking is the end product.

On first blush, Rado's point of view is appealing. Anyone who has dealt intimately with individual schizophrenic patients through the course of their illness is more impressed by their strange feeling responses to the world than by almost any other facet of their behavior. The abject misery which they suffer all day long every day of their lives is pathetic and gripping. The way in which they see the world as bleak and the way that they experience themselves as "the living dead" reminds one well of Rado's notions. Such schizophrenic feelings are often so poignant that the observer begins to wonder why any human beings choose to go on living. Presumably this dreaded desolation accounts for the many suicides among schizophrenic patients.

Is anhedonia a uniquely schizophrenic phenomenon? If given a choice of psychiatric illnesses in which to apply this designation, I would prefer to place anhedonia in the laps, or better in the minds, of depressed individuals. If there is any situation in which the primary difficulty is "inability to experience pleasure" this certainly should be mental depression. Indeed, mania and depression are traditionally called "the affective disorders." Anyone who has worked in a psychiatric hospital is familiar with the theme song of depressed patients, repeated by them over and over, interminably and often to the ultimate exasperation of the therapist, "Life is devoid of happiness for me . . . food has lost its taste . . . sex has no appeal . . . I don't care about my work. I don't care about anything . . . there can be no joy in life for me."

Surely anhedonia is more appropriate for these patients as a unique feature of their mental life than it is for schizophrenics. With schizophrenics it is much simpler to assume that the lack of appropriate feeling responses to the world is the result of a variety of other disturbances which make it so complex and painful to articulate themselves with their environment, to mesh their lives with lives of their fellow men, that whatever native spunk they may have begun with is exhausted in the Herculean task of staying alive in society. There is little if any energy left over for the luxury of "being happy."

6

Symptoms

The schizophrenic thinks and feels in a strange, lonely, other-worldly way. Fine, but psychiatrists, social workers, nurses, all the general public don't usually encounter directly the deep-down affect and conceptualizations of the schizophrenic, fascinating though they may be. Instead, all of us deal more with the surface manifestations, the patient's symptoms. How do we go about understanding the symptoms of schizophrenia?

Ambivalence

Bleuler felt that all the variegated symptoms and subtypes of schizophrenia flowed directly from disturbances in the "simple psychic functions" of forming mental associations and experiencing feeling states of "affectivity." Symptoms of schizophrenia which are direct products of these disturbances were to be labeled "fundamental symptoms." The enormous ambivalence evident in the thinking and feeling of schizophrenics is an excellent example of such a symptom. Someone's thinking is presumably ambivalent when he expresses essentially opposite ideas in close juxtaposition. Bleuler described many examples, for instance: "I am Doctor H.; I am not Doctor H. . . . I am a human being like yourself even though I am not a human being." One of his patients described what was going on in his mind under these conditions, "[W]hen one expresses a thought, one always sees the counterthought. This intensifies itself and becomes so rapid that one doesn't really know which was the first."

If one gets to know a patient well it is evident that much of this seemingly meaningless intellectual ambivalence, this constant outpouring of contradictory statements, is quite meaningful. Sometimes the apparent ambivalence is a red herring. The patient is almost deliberately trying to confuse the doctor, holding him at arm's length, testing to see if he is dangerous or to be trusted. In these cases the ambivalent language is being used not so much to communicate but as a device to preserve the patient's sense of security, as Harry Stack Sullivan emphasized. The Scottish psychiatrist, Ronald Laing, sees these situations as expressing a conflict between the false outer self of the patient, which operates in accordance with the rules of the everyday world of other people, and the desires of the inner self, which lives in a world of fantasy divorced fully from reality. Since there is something of fantasy in all people, these ambivalent statements often take on a semblance of poetic and philosophical paradox. Laing has offered an entire volume of "ambivalent" aphorisms and poems.

His book, *Knots*, provides many eloquent commentaries on the existential dilemma of modern man, whether sane or schizophrenic. Examples abound: "They are not having fun . . . I can't have fun if they don't . . . If I get them to have fun, then I can have fun with them . . . Getting them to have fun, is not fun. It is hard work . . . How dare you have fun when Christ died on the cross for you! Was He having fun?"

Another example of the logical confusion and personal terror experienced most by schizophrenics but shared by all mankind is described by Laing in this way,

> Mother is cruel to me; but she is only being cruel to be kind because I thought she was cruel when she was cruel in punishing me because I was cruel to her to think she was cruel to me for punishing me for thinking she was cruel for punishing me for thinking . . .

Just as ambivalence may be intellectual, so it is often expressed in the realm of feelings. Bleuler provides many examples.

> The husband both loves and hates his wife. The patient's hallucinations reveal to the mother the longed for death of the child by the unloved husband. She breaks out in endless sobbing and moaning. She suffers the most intense anxiety that they are going to shoot her and yet she constantly begs the attendant to shoot her. She claims there is a black man outside her room. Then she breaks into a startling confusion of tearful demands, complaints and violence, demanding that she be kept in the hospital and permitted to join the black man, and constantly repeats "You devil, you angel, you devil, you angel."

Of course, it is hard to distinguish ambivalence of feeling from that of thinking. They usually go hand and hand. Bleuler, however, in the Swiss tradition of meticulous attention to detail and preoccupation with nuances of classification, attempted to differentiate yet other forms of ambivalence. For instance, he described ambivalence of "will" in speaking of patients who wanted to eat but at the same time did not want to eat. Such a patient would "bring the spoon to his mouth dozens of times but never complete the act." Another patient clamors for his release and then resists with much cursing when he is informed that he will be discharged; "he demands work only to become furious when something is given him to do and cannot decide to do the work."

It is quite likely that such mixed feelings about one's own volitions underline many stereotyped compulsive behaviors seen in schizophrenic patients. Patients may become obsessed with taking apart and then putting back together mechanical objects such as toys or even radios. The patient may for hours on end alternately pummel with his fist a picture of his mother and then kiss it. With chronic patients, these actions become reduced to simpler motor components so that, unless one knows how the behavior had first begun, its significance will be rather obscure. Thus, in the patient who began by striking and then kissing his mother's picture, these movements ultimately developed into a shorthand of clenching and opening his fist, but puckering his lips simultaneously with the opening of his fists.

Autism

Bleuler described numerous other symptoms in schizophrenia which seemed to derive from the initial disorders of association and affect but somewhat less directly than the ambivalence. He called these "compound functions." For instance, the overall way in which a patient relates to the outside world would be a compound function built up out of operations of the simple functions of thinking and feeling.

Bleuler viewed autism, the retreat from reality manifested by essentially all schizophrenic patients, as the most important disturbance of compound functions. Simply put, whether because they are unable to reason as most people do, or because they are devoid of normal human emotional responses or perhaps are cursed with an overabundance of them, schizophrenics have rejected the mundane real world. Instead they have retreated in their mental functioning to an inner life. Their behavior will be more or less bizarre and disjointed from reality depending largely on the extent to which they have divorced themselves from others and on how prolonged has been their sojourn away from meaningful contacts with other human beings. As a patient withdraws further and further, he loses the ability to distinguish between his fantasy life and the real world.

Perhaps this withdrawal is at the root of hallucinations. Since he can no longer tell the difference between his own thoughts and what people are speaking about in the immediate environment, he finds it all too easy to attribute his thoughts to forces or people outside of himself, and accordingly commences to "hear voices." Most psychiatrists would agree that, besides reflecting autistic withdrawal, hearing voices is a convenient device whereby the schizophrenic can renounce responsibility for his own ideas. In more chronic patients, things reach a point where, besides experiencing their own thoughts of hallucinations, they have difficulty discerning whether people who are speaking to them are real or simply hallucinated.

Hallucinations are the most flagrant and obvious of schizophrenic symptoms. Thus, when I'm called to interview a patient, I may find that after twenty minutes of discussion I am not really sure whether the individual is schizophrenic or "sane." The task of deciding whether someone is manifesting a "schizophrenic thought disorder" or "schizophrenic disturbance of affect" is really quite difficult. Many anxious, neurotic patients often have difficulty making themselves clear and may even seem incoherent, especially if they do not share your own socioeconomic and intellectual background. Similarly, many nonschizophrenics and even "normal" individuals converse with a seemingly blunted affect. The diagnosis is often solved by the simple expedient of asking, "Are you hearing any voices?" Or, hoping to avoid the patient's denying his hallucinations in order to avoid hospitalization, I might surprise him with "Just what are the voices telling you?" Often my efforts are rewarded with replies such as "They keep repeating to me, 'everything will be all right, everything will be all right, you will not be forsaken,'" bringing the diagnostic dilemma to a quick close. If hallucinations are so pathognomic, perhaps they should be viewed as the key disturbance in schizophrenia.

On the other hand, many unmistakably schizophrenic patients never hear voices. For this reason, Bleuler felt, and most modern psychiatrists would fully agree, that hallucinations, whether auditory or visual, whether of tactile sensations or even of smell, are not the "key disturbance" in schizophrenia. Bleuler did not even feel that they were as directly derived from the primary disorders of feeling and thinking as were ambivalence and autism, and hence did not look upon hallucinations as "fundamental symptoms" to the "four A's" of association, affect, ambivalence, and autism.

While the mnemonic of the four A's is the way most American psychiatrists have been coached in their techniques for diagnosing schizophrenia, Bleuler actually discussed other fundamental symptoms which followed upon the alterations in thinking and feeling. For instance, he pointed out the abnormality in the "will" of schizophrenics, something we have already touched upon in our discussion of ambivalence. Most patients don't seem to have very strong volition. Among the patients Bleuler encountered in Swiss psychiatric hospitals, many seemed to lack the initiative to do anything on their own, hence would become slovenly and neglect their personal habits until their rooms became an intolerable collection of odors of urine and smeared feces. But it would seem unfair to accuse schizophrenics of lacking volition. Clearly things are far more complicated. Once they are in a mental institution for a prolonged period, their situation is analogous to that of a convict with a sentence of life imprisonment and no hope of parole. Why bother? And whether or not they have been literally sentenced and serve a long period in a mental institution, the sentence of their emotional disease is an even more confining, bleak, and demoralizing one than that of the convicts sentenced to "life" or perhaps even to death.

Intact Intellect

Similarly, while Bleuler suggested that a seeming *dementia* or mental deterioration of schizophrenics

might be derived from alterations in feelings and thinking, he was quite circumspect about such a conclusion.
He felt quite strongly that Kraepelin and all the earlier
psychiatrists had been gravely in error in labeling
schizophrenia as a form of *dementia*. He was convinced
that *dementia* was rare even in chronic schizophrenics.
What looked like mental deterioration in schizophrenics
might be simply a result of the prolonged loss of
emotional link to the world. For us this seems obvious.
For Bleuler, his declarations of the nonexistence of a
pure *dementia* in schizophrenia amounted to something
of a revolution in psychiatric thought. For Bleuler it took
courage to say,

> In no other disease is the disturbance of intelligence more
> inadequately designated by the terms "dementia" and "im-
> becility" than in schizophrenia. We see absolutely nothing in
> this disease of "definitive loss of memory images" or other
> memory disturbances which properly belong to the concept
> of dementia. Thus . . . even the severest schizophrenics are
> not demented . . . dementia, in the sense of the organic
> psychoses, is something fundamentally different . . . it is of
> prime importance to establish that even in a very severe
> case of schizophrenia all the fundamental functions that are
> accessible to present tests are preserved. In mental defi-
> ciency complicated connections of ideas and associations
> are never formed; in organic cases much has been lost, if
> not by actual brain damage at least by the very poor
> utilization of the intellect. In contrast, even the most [ap-
> parently] "demented" schizophrenic can under proper con-
> ditions suddenly demonstrate productions of a rather highly
> integrated type such as cunning attempts at escape.

He emphasizes that, if the behavior or performance
on psychological tests of a schizophrenic are to be
viewed as demented, it is only in the very limited sense
that performance is impaired with respect to specific

situations, ones that carry with them emotional consequences. Thus the schizophrenic impairment in performance really reflects his failure to comply with the demands of the examiner.

In accordance with the fact that there is nothing fundamentally disturbed about the intellect of a schizophrenic patient, Bleuler astutely noted that other basic sensory and intellectual functions are not impaired. Thus while the patient may be hallucinating all day long, his visual and auditory acuity are quite intact. Though he may be babbling incoherently, his general intelligence and ability to solve complicated verbal or mathematical problems may be quite normal. Even while in a catatonic stupor, he is not really out of contact and is often quite alert, noting and remembering vividly every event in the environment. Woe to those physicians, nurses, and other hospital staff who forget this and carry on indiscrete conversations in the presence of some wildly crazy and seemingly out-of-contact patients. Not only are some patients alert and capable of being fully lucid, but they are also perfectly well oriented as to where they are and the date and time of day.

Bleuler made quite a fuss about the lack of disturbance of sensation, memory, and consciousness for several reasons. First of all, the preservation of these functions in schizophrenic patients was and still is a cardinal tool in distinguishing schizophrenics from individuals with organic psychoses, whether due to brain tumors, fever, drugs, or vitamin deficiencies. Nowadays, with the widespread abuse of psychotropic drugs, some of which are concocted in underground laboratories and not widely known to the medical profession, physicians frequently encounter patients who are psychotic and behave very much like schizophrenics. However, with most drug-induced psychoses there will be some disturbance in these simple mental functions. Quite often with drug psychoses patients will not be able to tell where they are. They will be confused or delirious and be genuinely unable to remember what happened in the preceding hours or days.

By contrast, a schizophrenic patient does not experience any of these difficulties. A subtle point, to which Bleuler addressed himself with vehemence, is that schizophrenics may often simulate disturbance in sensation and/or memory or cognition, either out of a willful attempt to deceive the physician or as a product of their psychotic thinking. Apparently, in nineteenth- and early twentieth-century psychiatry, schizophrenics were frequently not distinguished from patients with organic psychosis for these very reasons. Accordingly, Bleuler emphasized,

> Disturbances and defects [in sensation, memory, consciousness, and motility] are very often falsely diagnosed because the examiner and the patient do not really speak the same language. The patient takes symbolically what the physician understands in its literal sense. Thus a patient insisted that he could not see, that he was blind, while it was more than obvious that his eyesight was unimpaired. What he meant was that he did not perceive things, "as reality." A female patient insisted with the greatest firmness, in answer to the question as to how long she had been in the hospital, that she had only been there three days, although she had given many proofs of her normal orientation to time and had been in the institution for many weeks. This time period of "three days" was for her identical with "my whole life." She herself was able to give the explanation: that the "first day" corresponded to be one in her earliest youth when she had been morally delinquent; the "second day" corresponded to that when she had done the same thing as a grown-up young woman; the "third day" had not yet been brought to completion.

Bleuler looked upon this dissimulation as a form of "double-entry bookkeeping." "They know the real state of affairs as well as the falsified one and will answer according to the circumstances with one kind or the other type of orientation—or both together."

What Comes Second and What Comes First?
Accessory Symptoms

Recognizing that there can be individuals whose mental life is grossly disturbed without any true impairment of sensory perception, cognition, and intellect probably was the first key toward the realization that all such patients suffered from a single disease or collection of diseases. This separation of people suffering from "functional psychoses," i.e., crazy people with intact sensations and intellect from those with organic psychosis, took place sometime during the course of the nineteenth century. There was a delay of several decades, perhaps fifty or more years, before Emil Kraepelin unified the constellation of functional psychoses (other than manic depressive disease) as *dementia praecox* and another decade or so before Bleuler, with his concept of schizophrenia, made sense out of the great variety of disturbed behaviors manifested by these patients. Why the protracted lag before the dawning of the concept of schizophrenia? It seems so obvious to the contemporary psychiatric and even lay communities. Surely there could have been no lack of interest in these patients. The best estimates are that the incidence of schizophrenia has remained the same throughout history. Thus schizophrenic patients must have accounted for a massive number, perhaps even a majority, of all hospital beds in the nineteenth century.

The difficulty seems to have resided in the fact that what Bleuler calls the "accessory symptoms" of schizophrenia were so dramatic that they came to dominate the psychiatrist's impression of his patients. The principal accessory symptoms are hallucinations and delusions. As already mentioned, to the sane person, the notion of hearing a voice which is not there or seeing or feeling or smelling what is not present in the environment is remarkable and dominates the imagination. The excitement and stupor of a catatonic patient are spectacular. Similarly, the systematized delusions of the paranoid schizophrenic can be quite fascinating, frightening, and awesome to the observer, so that he may be less interested in other, more subtle disturbances of his patient's mental life.

These accessory symptoms influence one's thinking about schizophrenia in yet another way. People get committed to mental institutions because their behavior is grossly deviant one way or another from the conventions of society. Running around the house naked in a wildly excited state; lying rigid on the floor for days on end seemingly out of contact with the environment and at the same time letting one's urine and feces drip all about; announcing that God has spoken to you and annoints you as the savior of all mankind—these are "valid" reasons for hospitalizing someone. An individual can function reasonably smoothly in society even while his thinking and feeling are greatly impaired and his inner life is ensconced more and more in a world of fantasy. He can even have been hearing voices for years and years, yet be left at his liberty, unrecognized and free from the pens of those who wield mental commitment papers, provided that he minds his own business and doesn't tell too many people about the incredible things that are happening inside his head. Since schizophrenic individuals are by nature shy and withdrawn human beings, they will generally tend to remain well-behaved, despite their growing terror and disorganization.

If we agree with Bleuler that hallucinations, delu sions, and catatonic behavior are only "accessory," our net for the population of people who may be suffering from schizophrenia widens tremendously. A direct implication of Bleuler's thinking is that untold numbers of individuals, generally thought to be "all right" although rather shy, lonely, and perhaps a little peculiar, are very much schizophrenic but have simply not yet developed the more bizarre and recognizable stamps of the disease.

Although Bleuler predicted that there may exist many schizophrenics who function more or less adequately in society, it is only since the 1950s that labels have been affixed to these individuals. There are now a glut of categorizations. Such patients have been variously called pseudoneurotic schizophrenics, pseudopsychopathic schizophrenics, borderline schizophrenics, schizoid personality, stormy personality, and so on. The difficulty, of course, is that, insofar as these patients fail to display a full spectrum of schizophrenic behavior, it is difficult to be sure of the diagnosis.

The overly liberal application of the stamp of schizophrenia has made this situation, at least in the United States where diagnostic liberalism is most rampant, something of a travesty. Nonetheless, the fact that high rates of alcoholism, apparently psychopathic behavior, and other "borderline" behaviors tend to occur with astonishing frequency in the families of schizophrenic patients, tends to convince me that there is a large element of truth to the notion. The task lying before psychiatrists in the future will be to devise some fool-proof means of diagnosing these individuals who represent part of the "schizophrenia spectrum."

Clearly, schizophrenia in the absence of hallucinations and delusions is a tremendously important entity. But it is just as clear that such an entity poses intolerable burdens for the diagnostic acumen of psychiatrists. In the best of situations, psychiatrists are denied clear-cut biochemical tests of the sort that so simplify the life of the internist and surgeon. If psychiatrists were expected to make reliable, reproducible diagnoses of schizophrenia with no more other guide than their intuitive skills in sniffing out the "fundamental symptoms," they would never measure up to the task. Thus, the accessory symptoms form the major tools in the psychiatrist's diagnostic armamentarium, the bread and butter of the psychiatric craft. These accessory symptoms have always provided dramatic material for writers of fiction. Without the excitement and awe generated in the beholder of a schizophrenic manifesting these accessory symptoms, the world of the arts would be greatly impoverished. We would have to do without many great or not-so-great works of fiction, theatrical dramas, movies, and television soap operas.

Hallucinations

Most schizophrenic hallucinations are auditory. What schizophrenics usually hear are voices. In the most common type of hallucinations, voices threaten or condemn the patient, or almost as frequently console him. It is much rarer for patients to hear simple sounds, although these may presage the coming of full-fledged "voices," much like footsteps heralding an approaching stranger or friend. Why do schizophrenics so characteristically hear voices? Probably the hallucinations serve an important function in the patient's mental life. If the voices announce his impending doom, it may turn out that they reflect a wish or need of the patient to punish the "bad" part of himself. If the voice comforts, "It will be all right, it will be all right, it will be all right," it often seems that the patient is striving to pull himself together in the face of his galloping mental disintegration.

Seen in this way, hallucinations are ways of fulfilling healthier or sicker conscious or unconscious wishes of the patients. Thus, they remind one of the wish-fulfillment that Freud proposed as the major purpose for the dreams of normal people.

Patients' wishes vary enormously and their voices generally seem like some sort of attempt to control the environment, to make it come to terms with the patient in his turmoil, or better yet, to make that turmoil subside. Bleuler put it nicely when he said that

> the voices of our patients embody all their strivings and fears, and their entire transformed relationship to the external world . . . They are the means by which the megalomaniac realizes his wishes, the religiously preoccupied achieves his communication with God and the Angels; the depressed are threatened with every kind of catastrophe; the persecuted cursed night and day.

Because the hallucinations seem to serve these complex needs, it is easy to understand that illusions of simple sound, like tones or music, are uncommon. Moreover, some faint noise in the background, the sound of an air conditioner, leaves rustling in the breeze, which actually occur, are misinterpreted by the schizophrenic as having some enormous significance.

One can learn a great deal about the nature of thinking processes in schizophrenia by paying close attention to the contents of patients' hallucinations, "listening along with the schizophrenic." The voices embody all the characteristics of schizophrenic disturbances of feeling and thought. For example, we talked about extreme ambivalence as a striking phenomenon in schizophrenia. I can recall a patient hearing two voices in conversation. One constantly admonished, "You are damned!", while the other would counter "You are saved."

All these features of the voices heard by schizophrenics go along nicely with the notion that the voices are strictly the patient's own thoughts, which he has chosen, presumably without conscious awareness, to project onto the outside world. No one has any idea just how and why this projection takes place. A simple way of thinking about it is to suppose that by dint of his hallucinations the schizophrenic need no longer take responsibility for his own unbearable mental processes.

With patients early in their disease one can see the beginnings of this transformation of thoughts into voices. These individuals often report that they are hearing their own thoughts. They may complain, "I seem to be talking to myself more than ever." Gradually genuine hallucinations develop as the individual transfers the onus for his ideas from himself onto something outside himself, such as "The telephone lines take up all my thoughts."

Catatonic symptoms, the bizarre postures, stupor, and excitement, are included by many psychiatrists together with hallucinations and delusions as among prominent "accessory symptoms." Hallucinations and delusions occur in all the different subtypes of schizophrenia. While most schizophrenic patients can display some catatonic manifestations, these are generally looked on as being associated specifically with the catatonic form of schizophrenia and are best discussed there.

Delusions

Just as hallucinations may begin uneventfully as a somewhat worse case of talking to one's self than is experienced by normal people, so do delusions make their appearance insidiously. Delusions are the hallmark of paranoid schizophrenics but occur in other forms of the disease as well. People with paranoid schizophrenia in their future often are naturally suspicious and worrisome types. They misinterpret every criticism as conveying malevolent intent. These are the people who love to argue (if they are in fact capable of love at all) and are eager to leap into a lawsuit at the slightest provocation.

It is important to bear in mind that the majority of such "paranoid personalities" never do become schizophrenic. In fact, it is possible that a paranoid temperament is not directly related to schizophrenia in any fashion. According to this way of thinking, paranoid schizophrenia is simply schizophrenia which happens to occur in a person who coincidentally has a paranoid disposition. Conversely, many paranoid schizophrenics were not particularly litiginous, argumentative, or in any way paranoid in their preschizophrenic life.

Another caveat cautions against labeling as paranoid schizophrenic all incipient schizophrenics who suffer from delusions. Most schizophrenics experience delusions early in their illness. Indeed some psychiatrists describe a kind of "primary delusion" which they feel to be a major symptom of schizophrenia. By this they mean a feeling that everything transpiring in the world has some special significance for oneself. The patient cannot put a label on it. He doesn't feel that anyone is against him, nor does he have any grandiose conception of his own position in the world. It is a feeling of great awe. The patient feels that his state of self-awareness is greatly enhanced. He may be greatly elated by these seemingly incredible happenings or terrified that they presage imminent catastrophe. One psychiatrist described it this way: "He [the patient] is stirred to the death by some lines of the newspaper; he knows that they are of great significance for the state of the world and for humanity, but is unable to say what they indicate or whether they augur good or ill."

The primary delusions become transformed into more conventional delusions as the patient searches for a means to "explain" his breakthrough of awareness: "I went into a café and there were three white tables; it seemed to me that this might mean the end of the world." Interestingly, descriptions of primary delusions sound very much like typical psychedelic experiences under the influence of LSD or similar drugs.

Whatever the process, in many patients, and especially in paranoid schizophrenics, the primary delusion then undergoes "delusional misinterpretations" into what psychiatrists call "systematized delusions." Most people are familiar with the stereotyped delusions of "plots against me by the FBI," which is a typical delusion of persecution; or delusions of grandeur such as, "Of course, I am Jesus and will surely save you." The exact content of the delusions vary with the historical setting. In the nineteenth century, hospitals were literally filled with men walking about with one hand across the chest, believing themselves to be Napoleon Bonaparte. In the District of Columbia General Hospital, one can fill a ward at any given time with "the White House contingent," patients who were picked up attempting to scale the fence surrounding the White House because "I am here bearing an important message for the President."

Much more subtle are delusions of hypochondriasis. Innumerable patients, never known to psychiatrists, visit one doctor after another with various complaints. Every internist or general practitioner has his gallery of "crocks" who suffer from various imaginary illnesses and frequently compose as much as a third of his practice. The only way to tell the difference between these individuals, who may manifest few if any other symptoms, and a not-so-mentally-ill run-of-the-mill hypochondriac is by the tendency of the physical complaints of the schizophrenic to become somewhat bizarre. A patient may complain of a backache. Only on careful questioning does one appreciate his vague conviction that the bones in his back are turning to liquid.

Much as was the case with hallucinations, delusional thinking often mirrors the typically schizophrenic thought disorder. Details of the delusional system may not be connected logically but in a vague, tangential, "nonabstract" fashion. The delusions may harbor mutually contradictory ideas, reflecting opposing feelings, and in this way convey information about the profound emotional ambivalence of the patient. By contrast, many paranoid schizophrenics sport extraordinarily well-organized, logical, and seemingly coherent delusional systems. They may seem so sensible that one feels he is conversing with a very articulate gentleman who is intent upon an important and urgent issue.

7

Varieties

Few conceptual dilemmas bother the conventional medical specialist. If a patient has a fever, a cough and pain in his chest, the physician takes chest X-rays. Characteristic patterns in the film establish the diagnosis of pneumonia. The physician then wants to classify the pneumonia into one of its varieties, depending on the germ at fault, because this may have bearing upon the appropriate treatment. He asks the patient to cough vigorously, then places the sputum in an appropriate solution and waits for the offending bug to grow out. If small, round bacteria in a particular pattern and giving certain chemical reactions appear on the culture plate, he knows that the condition was caused by the *pneumococcus* and accordingly labels his patient with the diagnosis of pneumococcal pneumonia. If the patient's blood has antibodies to the Coxsackie virus, it is apparent that he is suffering from viral pneumonia of the Coxsackie type.

Things are not so simple for the psychiatrist. Through careful clinical observations over the years and more recently because of rigorous genetic studies, we can affirm that there does exist a disease called schizophrenia. But when it comes to classifying different types of schizophrenia, our task becomes almost insuperable. American psychiatrists often don't even bother to classify their patients, reasoning, why bother with all that effort when it really makes little difference as to how the patient is going to be treated and isn't particularly valuable in helping to predict a clinical course?

However, schizophrenia is the most important of the mental illnesses, both in terms of degrees of disruption of normal living and the theoretical importance for understanding the basis of normal and abnormal emotional functioning. Thus it is rather hard for the scholars of psychiatry to ignore the challenge of attempting to make sense out of the motley assortment of schizophrenic modes of life. And where there are no known causative bacterial agents to be cultured, no recognized biochemical abnormalities, one is left with the armchair task of dissecting different forms of the disease and making new taxonomies.

The classical subtypes of schizophrenia in all the textbooks since Bleuler are really collections of fairly clearcut symptoms which tend to go along together in some patients. Historically, each of these "symptom complexes" was labeled as a specific disease entity. But many patients who start off with one cluster of symptoms will drop them over a period of time in favor of another cluster, representing a different subtype of schizophrenia. Thus a single patient may at one time or another appear to suffer from all of the subtypes. Because of this interchangeability, Emil Kraepelin realized that they all must be part of the same disease. Nowadays, these subdivisions are still recognized as "official" diagnoses, largely because they are a convenient shorthand for describing the individual's behavior at the time of the diagnosis. The four major types which are recognized today are the same as those described by Bleuler. They are catatonic, hebephrenic, paranoid, and simple schizophrenia.

A. Catatonia

All the symptoms of catatonia were tied together as an entity coined by Kahlbaum in 1874. The word "catatonia" comes from Greek and means "tension." This is an apt description, because the most striking features of catatonic schizophrenia are the changes in the tension of the voluntary muscles.

When the layman speaks of catatonia he usually is thinking of the stuporous phase. In catatonic stupor, the patient looks like he is completely out of contact with reality. In point of fact, when such persons recover they often can prove to you that they registered everything that was going on about them with great accuracy even during the depth of their stupor. The "tension" of their muscles is involved in their capacity to adopt strange statuelike postures and maintain them for long periods of time. Some of these postures seem to defy gravity and could not possibly be assumed by any normal individual, with the possible exception of experienced yogis. While in these bizarre postures, an observer may move the patient's limbs to new positions, which he will maintain even after the examiner removes his hands, a peculiar phenomenon called "waxy flexibility." The ability of catatonic schizophrenics to treat their bodies like machines is manifested in other aspects of their behavior. They will obey orders literally like a robot. At the height of their immobility, catatonics will refuse to eat and lose (or perhaps truly give up) control of their bladder and bowels. In the back wards of large hospitals, such patients quite literally starve to death.

Yet catatonic patients can surprise the observer by emerging suddenly from a stupor of weeks or months duration to be completely lucid. It is as if they had suddenly "awakened." They may remain "awake" permanently thereafter, for catatonic schizophrenia is the form in which spontaneous recoveries are most frequent. Alternatively, the lucid period is brief, and the patient returns rapidly into his stupor.

At the opposite pole is the wild, frantic, catatonic excitement. Patients will suddenly run about, jump over furniture, bang on the wall and on the floor, cry, sing, scream, laugh, and do all these things at such a furious rate and with such rapid alternation between activities that it seems as if they are all taking place simultaneously. This behavior reminds the observer of many manic patients. The difference is that a manic person appears in much better contact with his environment. His activities can be comprehended fairly readily and may even appear quite clever. The manic is in some emotional contact with his environment. He emanates a feeling of aliveness. By contrast, even when hyperactive, the catatonic schizophrenic gives off the same aura of death-in-life as when he is stuporous. The excitement may alternate with stupor, and the interchange may be so rapid that observers become confused. Catatonic excitement takes on an especially frightening aspect when we realize that many such patients have actually run themselves to death from exhaustion and heart failure.

B. Paranoid Schizophrenia

In paranoid schizophrenia delusions of persecution or grandeur come to dominate the patient's life. In keeping with most medical tradition, the word paranoia, like catatonia, derives from Greek words which mean "resembling the mind." This refers to paranoid delusions which, in their better-formulated forms, can mimic rational, very complicated thinking. Because they use intellectual mechanisms in their symptoms, paranoid schizophrenics tend to preserve their intellectual functioning better than most schizophrenics. Also, paranoids tend to have been more intelligent prior to the onset of their illness than were other schizophrenics.

Because paranoid schizophrenics so frequently wrap their delusional systems into neat little conceptual packages, it may be difficult to prove that they suffer from the classically schizophrenic disordered thinking patterns. Many of the better-organized patients can go on for many years with a life style which appears perfectly normal, staying married and gainfully employed. The only difficulty is that "when scratched" one finds close to the forefront of their daily interests some complicated delusional system.

Such patients can be puzzling to their families. They seem to be mentally normal yet it is clear that they harbor "crazy thoughts." One patient of mine, Mrs. A., was an attractive forty-eight-year-old housewife, mother of two lovely young married daughters, with a devoted husband and stable marriage and life situation. She was the model housewife, keeping the home immaculate, active in community affairs, and having her daughters and son-in-laws and grandchildren over frequently for dinner.

But she complained that she was being left out of family life and people were keeping secrets from her. At first her husband assumed that she was a little concerned over the fact that the two daughters were much more spontaneously affectionate with their father than with their somewhat uptight, strict, and distant mother. Only after a year did it become apparent that the difficulty was more serious. She was not just being left out emotionally. She was confident that everyone else in the family had hearing devices which allowed them to find out just "what was going on" in the world. Her husband bought her a transistor radio. But it was clear that this was not what she wanted. She was finally hospitalized after she began hanging sheets over the windows to make sure that other people could not listen in with their devices.

Over a period of months, following a treatment program aimed at systematically ignoring her delusions, the "crazy" ideas gradually seemed to fade away. At least she did not talk about them anymore. But from some subtly suspicious glances and words which she let slip every now and then, I feel that more than a year afterwards, when "totally rehabilitated," she still was convinced of her delusions but had no intention of telling anyone about them lest they lock her up again in some mental hospital. At this time she had gone back to life as a typical housewife, a good member of the community, and present-bearing, if not overly warm, grandmother.

For Kraepelin, Mrs. A would certainly would not qualify for a designation of *dementia praecox.* She never showed the faintest hint of deteriorating, and her illness came on about the time of menopause rather than during adolescence. Kraepelin set up a separate category for people like Mrs. A. called paranoia, outside the boundaries of *dementia praecox.*

There are other individuals whose false beliefs are not so intricate and extensive as in pure paranoia yet not so bizarre and fragmented as with most paranoid schizophrenics. For these patients, whose condition usually lasts only for a brief period of weeks or months, psychiatrists have evolved the label of "paranoid state."

Both with paranoia and paranoid state, it is likely that there is a reasonable amount of schizophrenic thinking. Many patients thought to have pure paranoia, when followed over a period of several years, gradually change into what most observers would agree are bona fide paranoid schizophrenics.

C. Hebephrenia

Hebe was the adolescent daughter of Zeus and Hera of Greek mythology. By vocation she was the cup-bearer to the gods. It is said that she was something of a lush—not that she drank too much, but that she could not hold her liquor. Moreover, she was not the most reliable of employees. Often she would sip some of the wine she was supposed to be carrying to the gods. Thereupon she would become quite silly, giggling in a childlike, embarrassing, showoff fashion, a little like a clown. The German psychiatrist Hecker in 1871 appropriated her name to describe what he thought to be a

unique psychosis characterized by silly, clowning behavior with shallow feeling, grimacing, and manneristic
behavior. The dialogue of Hecker's patients was sprin-
kled with apparently meaningless new words, "neolo-
gisms." They would become hung up on the last words
of sentences to which they would affix rhyming sounds,
e.g., "I hate you, blue, glue, clue." Hecker called this
disease hebephrenia.

Unfortunately, there is nothing at all funny about
people with hebephrenia. Like many circus clowns and
too many people we know who behave in everyday life
like clowns, their behavior is far more pathetic than
amusing. When they speak in rhymes, and link phrases
because of similarity of sound rather than of concept,
this is no joke. These are the patients with the most
severe disturbance of thinking of any schizophrenics.
They display Bleuler's abnormality of mental associations with consummate fidelity. Nothing could be more
"concrete" than to have difficulty finishing a sentence,
getting caught up in the middle of some of their "clang"
associations, in which they keep on spewing out words
that sound alike. For instance, "I came to the hospital to
play, gay, way, lay, day, bray, donkey, monkey." As
thinking patterns deteriorate, the speech of hebephrenic individuals becomes incoherent, a jumbled mass of
unrelated words, which psychiatrists have labeled
"word salad."

Hebephrenic schizophrenia most often appears slowly and insidiously during adolescence. The patients tend
to go downhill more than most other schizophrenics.

Hecker, of course, was wrong. Hebephrenia is not a
unique disease, but merely one symptom cluster within
the general class of schizophrenia. If one follows hebephrenic patients, often they will change their pattern of

symptoms and come to resemble other forms of schizophrenia. Moreover, the reverse pattern is even more frequent. Patients who were first paranoid or catatonic will sometimes come to take on many typically hebephrenic behaviors. This is usually a bad sign, foreboding a downhill course.

D. Simple Schizophrenia

In terms of variety and richness of symptoms, simple schizophrenia is indeed the "simplest" of the schizophrenias. What is most characteristic about the behavior of simple schizophrenics is the sheer absence of behavior. These people do little to distress others. They are the most inconspicuous human beings imaginable. They never make waves.

Gradually one detects an impoverishment of their intellectual and emotional life. Their relationships with other people, never particularly abundant, dwindle to nonexistence. It is generally impossible to discern exactly which events might have precipitated an emotional disorder. Quietly, they slide into a world devoid of contact with reality while losing interest in school, family, and job. In talking with these patients, one is hard pressed to elicit anything bizarre. They may hear voices, but often are unable or do not wish to talk about them. They rarely sport any bizarre, spectacular delusions of persecution or grandeur. All of them unquestionably display the typically schizophrenic, vague, tangential way of thinking. However, because their thoughts are so limited in scope and impoverished in content, one finds it difficult to pin down the thought disorder.

Bleuler foresaw an extremely important implication

of the simple schizophrenic's pattern of "non-symptoms." He fully appreciated that people are labeled as mentally ill and hospitalized whenever and only insofar as they bother other people. Simple schizophrenics are extremely inoffensive people. Accordingly, the great majority of them are not in mental institutions but live on the fringes of society. Many exist as hoboes, quiet alcoholics, prostitutes, and, in the past decade, as hangers-on in hippie communities. For these are the life styles in which it is often fashionable to lack any commitment to life. By moving about from place to place, especially in bohemian sorts of groups, it is possible to be part of a community without genuinely participating. Becoming a Skid Row alcoholic is almost an ideal solution for the simple schizophrenic. It affords a loose network of pseudofriends, and, at the same time, being inebriated is an efficient means of rationalizing and making more bearable a lack of contact with other people.

In Bleuler's day there were no private psychiatrists doing psychotherapy with vaguely neurotic people at such-and-such-many dollars per hour. Almost all psychiatry was focused within mental hospitals. From the point of view of "mental hospital psychiatry," simple schizophrenia was one of the rarest forms. However, in terms of the total number of people with schizophrenia, it is possible that this may well be an extraordinarily prevalent condition in life. Perhaps many individuals who continue to function in society, stay married, have jobs, but do so always on the borderline of "dropping out" are in fact simple schizophrenics whose disorder is relatively mild, or who have been held together and kept functioning by strong positive social and family influences.

A Happy or Sad End

For many years psychiatrists have noticed certain differences between schizophrenics who tended to get better quickly and those who had a poor outcome, spending the rest of their lives in mental hospitals. Some of these differences in the life style of diverse patients before their schizophrenia first makes its appearance seem related to the ultimate course of the illness. Specifically, patients who have functioned fairly normally before developing schizophrenia tend to do far better than those who have always, since their mother's earliest recollections, been rather strange and withdrawn. Also, those patients with the seemingly healthy life style before their mental breakdown tend to enter a schizophrenic state suddenly after some clearcut precipitating event, while those who had always been withdrawn ease slowly and insidiously into progressive isolation from other people. One widely used designation for these two types is "reactive" and "process" schizophrenia respectively.

Process schizophrenics are individuals whose personality was always lacking in integration. Their families can verify that since earliest childhood they were inadequate in relating to other children. In adolescence they failed to develop socially. They never were able to find an appropriate vocation. Their responses to events about them were invariably strangely blunted, almost absent. Beginning in late adolescence they withdraw more and more from daily activities, become apathetic and indifferent and often commence to have strange thoughts about their bodies, which are assumed by others simply to represent hypochondriac ruminations. When it finally becomes clear that they are thinking in queer, bizarre ways, they may be hospitalized. Invariably there are no obvious environmental reasons for their breakdown.

Process schizophrenics have the gloomiest prospects for recovery. They are called process schizophrenics, because they provide convincing, if terribly sad, evidence for Emil Kraepelin's concept of an inherent schizophrenic process which starts early in life and runs its tragic course regardless of all the heroic therapeutic efforts of physicians.

By contrast "reactive schizophrenics" seem to have developed their disease in "reaction" to some severe and obvious external stress. Careful review of their early years as infants and small children shows no major abnormalities. Their physical health was good. Both at home and at school they got along reasonably well. In adolescence they developed acceptable relationships with the opposite sex and had numerous friends.

Whereas the process schizophrenic lapsed into his psychosis with a "whimper," his reactive confrere goes crazy with a great big bang. Instead of gradual withdrawal, reactive schizophrenics usually have florid symptoms with vivid hallucinations, many ideas of reference (thinking that everything going on about them applies to themselves), and vague feelings that people are out to get them. Many patients who begin with catatonic symptoms, especially catatonic excitement, fall into the category of reactive schizophrenia are by definition process schizophrenics, as are many hebephrenics.

While classification according to symptoms—catatonic, hebephrenic, paranoid, simple—gives us much of the flavor of the sorts of people one sees walking about mental institutions, the process–reactive dichotomy possesses the utility which Kraepelin sought in developing the concept of *dementia praecox,* namely, the ability to predict. Prediction is enormously important from the very practical view of helping the families of patients know what to expect in ensuing years. And being able to predict anything at all gives psychiatry a big boost toward becoming more of science than of art or craft.

Many European psychiatrists do not rest easy with the description of process and reactive schizophrenia. They are still influenced by the doctrine of Kraepelin that schizophrenia is to be equated with *dementia praecox.* Accordingly all that is schizophrenia must deteriorate, and what does not deteriorate is not schizophrenia. Like the Americans they too recognize that many patients with typically schizophrenic patterns of behavior are capable of recovering to full normality with no evidence of residual thought disorder. To deal with these nasty exceptions to the rule of schizophrenia deterioration, they have invented the term "schizophreniform" to describe most of the patients we have characterized as reactive schizophrenics. At first glance one might think the European psychiatrists rather rigid to insist that reactive schizophrenics, despite their displaying typically schizophrenic symptoms, don't suffer from the "disease" of schizophrenia simply because they fail to deteriorate. But recent genetic evidence suggests that perhaps they are right in maintaining that schizophreniform psychosis is quite distinct from schizophrenia. Schizophrenia occurs frequently in the relatives of adopted children who are ill with "true [process] schizophrenia." However, the relatives of adoptees who become "reactive schizophrenics" sport no such taint. There is no more likelihood of schizophrenia occurring in these families than is the case for control families. This suggests that process schizophrenia is an inherited disease while reactive schizophrenia may not be genetically determined.

These differences in psychiatric nomenclature, which vary tremendously as one steps across national boundaries, can often be confusing. In the United States the term schizophrenia is applied to a large number of patients, perhaps too many, some of whom do poorly and some of whom do well. In most of continental Europe, on the other hand, if someone is referred to as suffering from true schizophrenia, you can be sure that he is in the throes of a very grave illness which may last for a long time, should he recover at all.

Another widely used appellation in psychiatry is "acute" as opposed to "chronic" schizophrenia. Acute schizophrenics are those whose illness comes on suddenly and hence are often the same patients as reactive schizophrenics. Chronic is usually taken to mean both that the illness appeared gradually and that it has lasted a long time. Hence chronic schizophrenia applies largely to process patients. These distinctions are by means foolproof. Process schizophrenics may experience a number of acute episodes during their life history. Some patients with a healthy adjustment before illness will go on to deteriorate and never leave the mental hospital. Some schizophrenics with a favorable outcome begin their illness in a gradual rather than an acute fashion.

Is Everybody Crazy? The American Diseases:
Pseudoneurotic and Borderline Schizophrenia

American psychiatry has been dominated, far more than psychiatry in other parts of the world, by psychoanalysis. The great virtue of the psychoanalytic influence in American psychiatry is that emphasis is placed upon lengthy, intensive interviews designed to elicit feelings and thoughts which would otherwise be hidden below the surface. Under the relentless probing of the psychoanalytically oriented interviewer's subtle questions and diligent listening, all manner of distorted lustings and terrors are unearthed, even from mildly neurotic or normal individuals. Like the "third degree" techniques of police interviewers, or perhaps even more like the brainwashing technology of Russian and Chinese jailers, the psychiatrist's probing of his patients' unconscious mental functioning can often crack through the surface and let loose floods of crazy-sounding verbiage.

Perhaps it is for this reason that American psychiatrists see schizophrenia lurking behind a façade of normality and neurosis in vast numbers of patients. Whatever the reason, there is little doubt that Americans have greatly widened the umbrella of schizophrenia to include so many different patients that at times the diagnosis becomes meaningless.

Of course, they have erected diagnostic edifices and classification systems to deal with this morass. Thus patients who would not fit the criteria for schizophrenia if strictly defined by European standards, but who are revealed by careful interview to be thinking a little "loosely," have been called pseudoneurotic or pseudopsychopathic schizophrenics, depending on whether their overt symptoms are of neurosis or psychopath. Others who are not definitely neurotic or psychopathic are called "borderline." We should explore these entities, because if these conditions do reflect meaningful forms of schizophrenia, then the social implications are considerable.

Pseudoneurotic schizophrenia was first described

by Paul Hoch and Philip Polatin in 1949. A number of their patients were extremely anxious and severely neurotic, had little pleasure in life, and failed to improve much with psychoanalytically oriented psychotherapy. Their thinking processes seemed somewhat fuzzier than those of most neurotic patients. Because of the severe neurotic symptoms, failure to respond to treatment, and aberrant thinking patterns, Hoch and Polantin labeled them as pseudoneurotic schizophrenics.

If one believes strongly that neurotic symptoms must invariably succumb to the ministrations of a skilled psychotherapist, then it would be easy to conclude that a neurotic who does not recover with psychotherapy must not really have been neurotic. In retribution for his failure to comply with vigorously administered doses of psychotherapy, the recalcitrant fellow is reclassified as schizophrenic.

I doubt that it is fair to critize Hoch and Polatin so strongly for the concept of pseudoneurotic schizophrenia. In truth, they felt that they were dealing with people whose neurosis was considerably more severe than the usual sort of patient. Their patients had a "pan-neurosis," by which they meant that the patients had innumerable neurotic complaints, including obsessional thoughts, compulsive acts, phobias, hysterical symptoms, hypochondriasis, and vague depression. They could not concentrate well and sometimes felt weird and unreal.

In addition, these individuals suffered from "pan-anxiety." They were anxious about everything they were involved in. On meeting friends at a party their palms would sweat and they would feel a choking-up sensation. At work they became anxious and their hearts would palpitate. Sexual encounters were loaded with anxiety for them.

With such difficulty in everyday living, it is no wonder that they failed ever to have any fun or to experience even the smallest pleasures of life, and accordingly therefore suffered from anhedonia. Nothing in life held great appeal or would produce more than a brief satisfaction.

None of these patients were obviously schizophrenic. Their thinking was generally cogent. They did relate to other people. However, in unstructured psychoanalytically oriented free association sessions, Hoch and Polatin felt that the things they said were a little "loose." Similarly, some of their responses in the Rorschach tests or when interviewed under the influence of sodium amytal, "truth serum," were vague and tangential.

The concept of pseudoneurotic schizophrenia has become reasonably popular in the United States. As many as a third to half of patients entering certain psychiatric clinics are thus pigeonholed. Is this fair? Perhaps it would be simpler to assume, as do European psychiatrists, that these are simply patients with particularly severe pervasive neurosis.

To resolve this question, it would be nice to know whether or not there is a genetic susceptibility for developing pseudoneurotic schizophrenia or whether, as Kety had found for reactive schizophrenia, it is not genetically determined.

Like the pseudoneurotic category, pseudopsychopathic schizophrenia is a poorly characterized entity. These are patients who appear to be psychopathic, that is, to behave antisocially. Such individuals are often involved in crimes like larceny, bigamy, assault. As children they were truants from school. Frequently they become addicted to drugs or alcohol. What is most striking about them is that while on the surface they may seem tough, defiant, sneering, and nonchalant, when examined closely it is evident that they are extremely anxious, filled with guilt, compulsive, and hypochondrical. Like the pseudoneurotic individuals, these patients do not display obvious schizophrenic symptoms so that the psychiatrist arrives at a diagnosis of schizophrenia only by inference.

Sometimes, when confined, pseudopsychopathic schizophrenics become overtly psychotic. The psychoanalytic way of viewing this situation is something like the following: Normally patients' antisocial behavior is a way of "acting out" their deepest conflicts and fears, so that, unlike neurotic individuals, they need not experience them. Thus, at lease superficially, they do not suffer the pangs of anxiety which so cripple the neurotic individual. When confined, as when in jail, or in the seclusion room of a mental hospital, they are forced to confront all the horrible feelings deep within them. This confrontation is so intolerably painful that they become frankly psychotic. Whether pseudopsychopathic schizophrenics (or "schizopaths," as they are often called) deserve to be designated schizophrenic is just as much an open question as is the case for pseudoneurotic schizophrenia.

"Borderline" individuals appear to possess some of the features both of pseudoneurotic and of pseudopsychopathic schizophrenia. They have many neurotic complaints, sometimes are antisocial in their behavior, sometimes are anxious, and at other times "act out" their anxiety by use of drugs or sexual perversions. While they seem quite sane during ordinary discourse, it is easy to elicit a tendency toward "schizzy" thinking by intensive exploration of their fantasy life or dreams. Such patients are attractive for the neophyte psychiatrist, because they appear to possess tremendous insight into their unconscious motivations and into links between their relationships with parents at very early ages and their present behavior. However, they rapidly evolve into exasperating patients as their unreliability becomes evident (especially by failure to keep appointments regularly and on time)—and when, after many months or years of therapy, the physician realizes that his patient is making no progress at all.

8

Making Sense of the Schizophrenic Mind

The task we set ourselves was to understand schizophrenia. Understanding something, in the best scientific sense, demands that one abstract from a motley assortment of disparate facts some unifying thread, some intellectual common denominator which will explain the whole morass of data. And to be really scientific, such an "understanding" ought to have predictive value so that one may test the hypothesis, confirm or reject it, modify it, make new findings, develop new technology, and so forth. In an area like psychiatry which is so lacking in hard facts, I am not sure that there is any possibility of adducing a truly heuristic theory of schizophrenia, much less one which will satisfactorily unify all the clinical findings.

What Comes First?

Bleuler's dogma held that what is primary in schizophrenia is a fragmentation of the "self," with attendant problems permeating all aspects of thinking and feeling. His theory was the first unifying hypothesis of schizophrenia and has not been much improved upon in the ensuing sixty or more years.

In the last few years there have been major breakthroughs in the treatment of schizophrenia and of other mental illnesses with drugs. And now it is becoming increasingly clear that the spinoff from these drugs as tools to further an understanding of brain function in the normal and diseased states may turn out to be of even greater importance than their utility in treating patients. But if the ever-accelerating accretions of understanding of brain chemistry and physiology are ever to bear fruit in solving the riddle of what goes on in the brains of schizophrenics, it would be well for psychological thinking about what is wrong in the "minds" of schizophrenics to move forward, and with good fortune, to mesh with the findings of the "harder" sciences.

Before attempting to formulate any global theories, we must get a few facts about schizophrenia straight or, at the very least, attempt to take some stance on certain major theoretical issues concerning the disease. First, is schizophrenia only one disease? Of course, as with most of these issues, there is no way of knowing for certain. However, the best evidence, derived especially from genetic studies, suggests that even if there are a group of schizophrenias, they must have something in common. For what tends to run in families is "schizophrenia" and not one of its subtypes. Within a given extended family one may find some members with paranoid schizophrenia, others with hebephrenic or catatonic forms of the disease. If we look at the process–reactive distinction, it is possible that there are different entities, since some of Dr. Kety's research suggests that reactive schizophrenia may not be familial. Another point favoring the existence of a single entity of schizophrenia is the fact that individual patients over the course of years will often switch subtypes.

Granted that there is some reasonably homogeneous disease entity corresponding to schizophrenia, how do we know that there is only a single brain abnormality? If the inheritance pattern obeyed some straightforward single-gene law of Mendelian genetics, one might argue that one gene must regulate some specific function which is impaired in the disease. Of course, it is also possible that, though a single gene may regulate a single chemical reaction, that chemical reaction may in turn influence several diverse psychological functions so that, even with a single chemical malfunction in schizophrenia, there would yet be a multiplicity of "fundamental" psychological abnormalities.

Unfortunately, in thinking about schizophrenia, we are spared the luxury of ruminating about such nuances. For the exact patterns of inheritance of tendencies to develop schizophrenia are by no means established. Though there may be only one abnormal gene, for all we know the disease might just as well involve a large number of genes which converge to form the right environment for developing schizophrenia.

Despite all these difficulties, or perhaps because of them, it may still be worthwhile to speculate about a single primary psychological abnormality in schizophrenia which might conceivably correspond to some aspect of brain function involved critically in the development of schizophrenic symptoms.

Many psychiatrists, psychologists, and neurophysiologists have put forth their special concepts of what might be fundamentally at fault in the mind of a schizophrenic person. All one need do is to detail the symptoms of schizophrenia and postulate that one "comes first" and then, by simple trains of logic, it is possible to deduce how the others might flow from the initial dysfunction.

A. THE NO FUN THEORY

For instance, the psychoanalyst Sandor Rado suggested that the primary abnormality is an inability to experience pleasure, "anhedonia." If nothing in life is fun, it is easy to imagine progressively withdrawing from most interactions with other people. Once one has disassociated himself from society, he will have little use for the tiring discipline of checking out every one of his thoughts for conformity with the real world but will instead prefer to amuse himself with his daydreams, his fantasy world. Soon, his thinking patterns will be sufficiently "private" that they will lack meaning for other people and will fail to follow simple rules of logic.

At this point the unfortunate chap will be the possessor of the typical schizophrenic thought disorder. For him to make sense out of the confusing array of other human beings, it will be necessary for him to develop accessory systems such as delusions and hallucinations. Thus anhedonia could readily serve as the common denominator of schizophrenic mental functioning.

B. TOO MUCH ANXIETY

But one could make the same argument for any of the other symptoms. Several writers have suggested that a very low threshold for anxiety, or a tendency to be overly aroused by any sort of stimulus, is fundamental to schizophrenia. If all life situations are anxiety laden, a person might well withdraw from reality, just as we have discussed for the individual who cannot experience pleasure. Again, all of the rest of the panorama of schizophrenia would follow in short order.

C. THE UNCONSCIOUS AWAKENS

Numerous psychoanalysts have been impressed by the facility with which schizophrenics can do what is excruciatingly difficult for neurotic patients, namely, they can all too easily bring their unconscious thoughts and wishes into conscious awareness. Since the unconscious mind, according to Freudian dogma, is filled with infantile lusts and terrors, its breaking through the barriers of repression and flooding the conscious mind with all manner of bizarre and perverted impulses could easily wreak havoc.

The thoughts of an infant, which purportedly compose a major portion of the unconscious mind, pay no heed to conventional subject–predicate logical thinking. Hence, if we assume that schizophrenics suffer first and foremost from an inability to repress unconscious mental contents, we could serve up the schizophrenic thought disorder forthwith.

D. THOUGHT DISORDER PRIMARY?

What if the thought disorder comes first? If you cannot think clearly, and instead reason all the time in a vague tangential fashion, you will surely experience the world differently from other people. Their motives will seem confusing, and you may mistakenly attribute ill-will to someone who has only your best interests at heart. In this way delusions will form. Since you cannot empathize with other peoples' feelings, you will tend to fear them, and your own feeling responses to the environment will be socially inappropriate. In terror of others you will withdraw. Here, too, we can easily imagine how all the symptoms of schizophrenia can emerge.

While all of these are plausible explanations, I have some reservations about each. The notion of attributing everything to an inability to experience pleasure does not quite fit for a number of reasons. One could never deny that future schizophrenics are notoriously unhappy individuals. Still, schizophrenics can experience the pleasures of intellectual and esthetic pursuits, even though they rarely delight in interpersonal relationships. Even more telling is the argument that, if any psychiatric patients suffer primarily from a deficit of pleasure, these are people with depression. Indeed, the inability to *enjoy* seems almost to be the essence of depression. But depressed people are not usually schizophrenic; and while schizophrenics may be depressed, it is a rather different thing from the depression of patients with classic manic depressive psychosis.

As for the anxiety hypothesis, it would seem that many neurotic individuals suffer from more anxiety than do a large number of schizophrenics. Often neurotics experience overwhelming anxiety, attaining the point of a state of terror and panic which a normal individual can hardly imagine. Of course, many schizophrenics who don't appear so anxious on the surface may well be suffering such terror and panic inside but have developed over the years remarkable skills at hiding their true feelings. Still, there appear to be many schizophrenics, especially simple schizophrenics, who probably have never known this sort of terror and whose anxiety quotient is probably exceeded by most anxious neurotics.

As tantalizing as is Bleuler's notion that the single fundamental abnormality in the mental functioning of schizophrenics is their inability to form appropriate "mental associations," it is too vague to satisfy our need for a "discrete" fundamental abnormality in schizophrenia. "Mental association" can mean almost anything. The linking together of two simple ideas to form a more complicated idea is a form of mental association. Pinning an appropriate feeling onto someone or something in the environment, such as "love" for "mother," is association. Reading the daily newspaper and recalling that the Richard Nixon visiting Communist China is the same Richard Nixon who was once an adamant anti-Communist is another type of association.

Even visual perception requires association. Everyone can recall times when they faintly detected the vague outline of a person in the distance and were able to fill in parts of the figure that they could not quite see and thus somehow recognize a dear friend. This is an important sort of mental association called perceptual integration. We fill in the gaps of what we do not see in complete detail.

Paying Too Much Attention to the Wrong Thing

Many researchers over the years have devised experiments to specify exactly what is impaired in the associational processes of the schizophrenic. Earlier we talked about the difficulty schizophrenics experience in interpreting proverbs, explaining them often in a too literal fashion. We mentioned the sorting tests in which schizophrenics grouped items together according to extraordinarily "concrete" categories, such as matching blocks only if they share an identical shade of blue rather than forming larger groups of blocks which are more or less bluish. Simply labeling the behavior of the schizophrenics as concrete or literal didn't seem to pinpoint anything specifically "schizophrenic," since people with organic brain damage showed similar abnormalities. By numerous variations on these earlier psychological tests as well as by many other types of experiments, subsequent workers have been able to define the schizophrenic abnormality a little more precisely. The general conclusion that has come out of a large number of such investigations is that the schizophrenic individual fails to abstract the general significance of issues with which he is confronted, because he pays too much attention to minor aspects of them and accordingly is distracted constantly. Thus, in sorting the blocks he may become distracted from the general notion of blueness by his fixation to the particular shade of one blue block. Accordingly his difficulty in sorting might be thought of as more "perceptual" than "conceptual."

The renowned psychologist David Shakow has spent many years developing psychological tests which so very clearly differentiate schizophrenic from nonschizophrenic people that there is no overlap between the groups. He began by measuring the reaction times of normals and chronic schizophrenic patients. In these experiments the subject is presented a warning signal to let him know that soon a tone will sound to which he must respond by pressing a button. The time between the warning signal and the tone to be responded to, called the "preparatory interval," is varied systematically. In general, schizophrenics have consistently slower reaction times than normal subjects. As the preparatory interval is lengthened, they do worse and worse. They are unable to take advantage of the warning which the preparatory interval provides, even when they know the exact amount of time between the warning signal and the tone to which they are supposed to tap the key. The schizophrenic patients just cannot maintain a state of readiness for responding to the test tone. Dr. Shakow feels that the failure to maintain a state of readiness occurs because the schizophrenics are constantly distracted by irrelevant aspects of the situation, either objects in the room or their own internal feelings. These distractions keep them from focusing on the tone.

This difficulty in focusing on the relevant aspects of a particular situation, this susceptibility to the influence of what is peripheral, seems to explain many other quirks of schizophrenic behavior in psychological experiments. For instance, in all sorts of test situations, schizophrenics don't become accustomed to stimulation but keep on responding with the same intensity to the twentieth presentation of a light or a noise, or a sexually arousing picture, as they did on the first presentation. They behave this way even though frequently their response to the first presentation was much weaker than that of a normal person. This is true not only in experiments in which the schizophrenics are required to answer or write something down or press a lever, but even when bodily reactions such as heart rate and electrical skin resistance are measured. For instance, when a painful stimulus is applied to a normal person, his heart rate accelerates markedly. However, when the same painful stimulus is applied again and again, the acceleration of the pulse is greatly attenuated. By contrast, the schizophrenic subject continues to show an accelerated pulse rate in response to pain even after many exposures.

After reviewing his own experimental findings over more than twenty years of research as well as those of many other scientists, David Shakow has become convinced that the common denominator to all of these schizophrenic performances is an "increased awareness of and preoccupation with the ordinarily disregarded details of existence—the details which normal people spontaneously forget, train themselves or get trained vigorously to disregard."

He feels that this is true from the earliest stages of schizophrenia to the most debilitated hospitalized chronic patient and is true for all of the different types of schizophrenic patients. He ties them all together with the metaphor,

> If there is any creature who can be accused of not seeing the forest for the trees, it is the schizophrenic. If he is of the paranoid persuasion, he sticks even more closely than the normal person to the path through the forest, examining each tree along the path, sometimes even each tree's leaves with meticulous detail. If at the other extreme he follows the hebephrenic pattern, then he acts as if there were no paths, for he strays off the obvious path entirely; he is attracted not only visually but even by smell and taste, by any and all trees and even the undergrowth and flora of the forest, in a superficial flirting, apparently forgetting in the meantime about the place he wants to get to.

All of this would be a description of how most chronic schizophrenics function in the world. By contrast, "The acute patient in the same forest undergoes a multitude of thrilling new experiences, reacting highly affectively, for instance, to new and unusual patterns of light on the leaves, or to novel and subtle patterns of form in the branches."

Maybe the World Looks Strange?

What Shakow is talking about sounds much more like a disturbance in integrating what the schizophrenic perceives in his environment rather than in his thinking *per se.* It is not that processes of thinking are first impaired but that the world is perceived in a disordered, jumbled fashion which is then reflected in the schizophrenic's thinking processes. It is like a computer gone wrong, not because the logical circuits are broken, but because of some malfunctioning in the "input" part of the machine.

If this sort of perceptual integration were primarily at fault in schizophrenics, we must remember that it would not be the same as a straightforward impairment of sensory perception. Vast numbers of studies of vision and hearing under all sorts of permutations of experimental conditions have shown that schizophrenics do not suffer failings in simple sensation. Instead, one would suppose that the abnormality lay in the way sensations were related to past memories and feelings before reaching the conscious attentive processes of the schizophrenic.

It is well known that how we perceive the world is not simply a function of our sense organs. The perception which reaches consciousness is not merely a point-for-point replica of what impinged upon the retina, the inner ear, or the sensory receptors in the skin, tongue, or nose. Instead, even in animals considerably lower than man there is a complicated process whereby sensations are transformed vastly before they reach awareness. And these transformations may vary enormously from person to person. A rose is a rose is a rose, but it is a very different rose to different viewers.

The *Gestalt* psychologists of the 1920s understood all this quite nicely. By means of a variety of simple experiments they demonstrated that our expectations influence how we perceive the environment. For instance, when the form of a triangle with substantial gaps in the sides is flashed on a screen for a brief interval, most people "fill in the gaps" and report seeing a complete triangle. There are many other well-known instances of how our feelings influence not only how we perceive things but also which items we will attend to and which we will disregard. Thus a sleeping mother continues to slumber peacefully while a parade of massive trucks lumbers noisily past her window. Yet she rouses almost instantly at the faintest whimper of her baby sleeping two rooms down the hall.

This tendency for internal mental states, memories, and emotions to influence what is perceived can be demonstrated directly by neurophysiological techniques. Drs. Hernandez-Peon and Michel Jouvet measured the electrical activity in the part of the cat's brain which is the first receiving station for auditory information. Whenever a sudden noise occurs, electrical activity appeared in this part of the brain. If cats were distracted from such noises by competing odors of fish or a jar of mice, the electrical response to the noise disappeared. As a consequence of these experiments, their view of how animals and people normally integrate what they perceive was that "attention involves the selective awareness of certain sensory messages with the simultaneous suppression of others . . . . During the attentive state it seems as though the brain integrates for consciousness only a limited amount of sensory information, specifically, those impulses concerned with the object of attention."

The fact that schizophrenics are unable to suppress perceiving irrelevant objects in their environment suggests that maybe their fundamental problem has to do with some sort of impairment of their brain's capacity to differentiate the important from the unimportant, and to discard whatever is not critical for the task at hand.

It is easy to imagine how a primary defect in perceptual integration could give rise to the whole spectrum of schizophrenic symptoms. Presumably this difficulty has been with the patient to a greater or lesser extent since his childhood. He sees and hears clearly. Yet he does not experience his visual and auditory sensations in quite the same way as his normal friends. Happenings which don't seem important and are shrugged off by the others impinge sharply and with no protective blunting upon the awareness of the future schizophrenic child. Small wonder that he becomes fearful of people and situations which are not at all frightening for most people.

Perception becomes extremely subjective in interpersonal relationships. We detect approval or rejection in the faintest wrinkle of our parents' face or the subtle modulation of their voices. It would be in the realm of communication with other people, especially parents and close family, to whom emotional ties are strongest, that misperception would be most rampant and beget misinterpretations over and over again.

These misinterpretations might represent the first phase of the schizophrenic thinking disorder. Distortions of thinking, as of perception, would display overinclusiveness and a failure to leave irrelevant, inconsequential elements out of one's thoughts. This sort of distracted, overinclusive thinking will of course appear to be excessively literal, concrete instead of abstract, and will fail to follow commonsense logic.

Similarly, misperceptions will wreak havoc in one's emotional life. By failing to modulate his perceptions appropriately, the future schizophrenic may continually be flooded with sensory input. As a consequence he may be overtly fearful, easy to panic, and thus behave or misbehave in strange ways in the classroom. Alternatively, he may shield himself from the perceptual onslaught and block out from emotional awareness the impact of his environment, especially the impact of the truly important people in his life. Thus, even at an early stage, he will turn off the world and turn his maladaptive perceptual antennae inward. In this way he will become preoccupied with his own internal fantasies which, though somewhat unpredictable, are certainly more under his control than the capricious external world.

He will soon appear to respond inappropriately to others, and will seem cold, aloof, unfeeling. This is not quite the same as a "lack of pleasure" or anhedonia. For there still is the capacity to experience pleasure, especially as a result of the patient's own fantasy life. Moreover, he can still appreciate and enjoy a beautiful piece of music or painting insofar as his attention holds to the esthetic qualities and avoids relating elements of the art object to his own past terrors.

Finally, as a stepchild of disordered perception, thinking, and feeling, there can emerge the secondary symptoms of schizophrenia, the delusions and hallucinations. Of course, if we assume that malfunctioning of perceptual integration is primary in the disease, we are in an especially good position to explain the genesis of hallucinations. This advantage may be particularly important. For hallucinations, hearing or seeing things which are not present in the environment, are probably the most "nonhuman" aspects of schizophrenics. Disorders of thinking and feeling are vague and hard to pin down. Unless they are quite bizarre, the presence of delusions does not enable one to label someone as "schizophrenic." All of us can recall episodes when we so misinterpreted the intentions of others and concocted such elaborate schemes to explain why someone was out to do us in that a suspicious observer might have thought us delusional. Hallucinations, on the other hand, clinch the diagnosis. Granted that hallucinations can occur in other conditions, with drugs or without drugs; still, nothing ever fully mimics the awe-filled, other-worldly aspect of a schizophrenic patient telling you about the voices he is hearing.

Even though all these experimental and clinical pieces of evidence favor the view that perceptual integration is more at fault in schizophrenia than other dysfunctions of the mental apparatus, we still must be cautious. In conjecturing about what goes on within the black box of our brains, we must beware of circular reasoning. It is almost impossible to discern with certainty just what *causes* what. The very fact that feelings and thoughts influence perception already suggests that underlying the disturbance in perceptual integration might be a more primary disorder of feeling or thinking.

The eminent psychopharmacologist Joel Elkes, in attempting to tie together brain mechanisms that regulate affect, perception, and cognition and which might be disturbed in schizophrenia, also favored a disruption of perceptual filters as the fundamental disorder in schizophrenia. But he could see how all these processes might interact so rapidly that a dysfunction of one would surely affect the others in short order and one would never be able to say which came first. He emphasized that the wish may thus become not only father to the thought but also to the image. In dim light, for example, the aggressive, destructive orally preoccupied schizophrenic will mistake his visiting wife for his much hated mother and viciously attack her; or savor blood in the roses which she brings him. In view of the promptness of these affective responses, the various stages of the operation must take place at very high speed.

First, All Is Frightening

Clearly we would benefit greatly from more evidence bearing on which block is loosest and slips first in bringing the whole toy castle of the schizophrenic psyche down with it. One ought to seek the loose block early in the game, before the whole spectrum of schizophrenic symptoms appear. We should be looking for the earliest detectable mental abnormalities in our quest to find the psychological failing at fault in schizophrenia. Ideally, one would like to study patients before they become schizophrenic. This extraordinarily difficult task has been undertaken by the psychologist Sarnoff Mednick.

Mednick sought out the children of chronic schizophrenic mothers, children who thus have a reasonably high chance of themselves becoming schizophrenic. He evaluated them by means of a battery of psychological tests when they were fifteen years old and had given no evidence of schizophrenic symptoms.

Five years later, twenty out of the original 200

children had suffered some sort of schizophreniclike decompensation. Mednick then went back to assess how they had differed in the testing five years before from the children who were still functioning reasonably well. There were several differences. For instance, the mothers of the "sick" subjects were more disturbed individuals than the mothers of the "well" ones.

Also, the two groups differed in the associations they gave to test words. In word association experiments, the experimenter states a word and asks the subject to say the first thing that comes to mind immediately, and to continue with new responses as one word suggests another. "Sick" subjects tended to drift away from the original stimulus word, so that after a series of associations they were producing words that were only dimly related to the original stimulus. This, of course, reminds one of the typically schizophrenic tangential way of thinking.

Of particular interest is how they responded in the galvanic skin response experiments. Galvanic skin response is a measure of the electrical activity of the skin, and is familiar to most people as the basis of "lie detector" tests. When one becomes anxious, nerves in the skin fire off, changing the electrical characteristics of the skin. In Mednick's experiments, the subjects' galvanic skin responses were "conditioned." Thus, these people were exposed to a loud and irritating noise which markedly altered the skin's electrical characteristics. Then the loud noise was paired with an innocuous tone of a particular frequency, the "conditioned stimulus." Soon the conditioning tone itself would elicit arousal as indicated by the galvanic skin response. Mednick wondered to what extent his subjects would generalize from one arousing, anxiety-laden situation to another. To assess the tendency to generalize, he then varied the pitch of the tone and determined just how much he had to change the pitch before the subject would no longer respond to it.

In comparison to the "well" group, the "sick" subjects responded to a considerably greater extent. Moreover, they tended to generalize much more than the "well" group. This is especially dramatic when one considers that these differences occurred years before the "sick" subjects decompensated and hence at a time when the experimenters did not notice any overt differences between their behavior and that of the more fortunate group.

Mednick concluded that the preschizophrenic, at an early stage, is hyperresponsive to environmental stimuli. He is easily aroused and becomes intensely anxious. Moreover, he overgeneralizes. If one teacher shouts at him, then he becomes panic-stricken when another teacher merely calls out his name in a quiet tone of voice. Indeed, interviews with the schoolteachers showed that the "sick" subjects tended to get upset easily. When upset or excited, their reaction persisted and they were not readily placated. Not surprisingly, though generally classified as "loners," the "sick" subjects were rated by their teachers as being very disturbing to the class.

Mednick felt that the schizophrenic thought disorder develops as a means of controlling the patient's tendency to become aroused and anxious by whatever he perceives going on about him. When confronted with what he sees as threatening, the preschizophrenic distracts himself by switching his attention to some unrelated thought which interrupts the emotional impact of the threat at hand. Thinking irrelevant thoughts as a means of avoiding frightening perceptions and ideas will soon eventuate in illogical and socially inappropriate thinking and behavior. This is how Mednick feels that schizophrenia evolves.

Of course, from his own experiments one might draw other conclusions. Mednick did find some suggestions of vague thinking in his "sick" subjects in the initial testing years before they decompensated. One might argue that the abnormal thinking begat the hyperarousal rather than vice versa. However, it is hard for me to understand how vague thinking processes of themselves would elicit hyperarousal to a noise. To the contrary, I would suspect that an individual who is incisive and attentive would be more susceptible to being startled by sudden, irritating noises. Thus I would tend to agree with Mednick that the vague thinking comes second, as a way of detoxifying the terror-laden world of the preschizophrenic.

Patients Say What They See

Yet another way of attacking the chicken-or-egg, what-came-first problem of schizophrenia is to explore in detail the earliest symptoms reported by patients undergoing a schizophrenic breakdown. Surprisingly, despite the voluminous amount of writing on this disease, there have been very few publications dealing with the earliest symptoms of schizophrenics.

A British psychiatrist, James Chapman, performed a particularly thorough study of such patients. He was impressed with the fact that schizophrenics experience profound changes in their perceptions and feelings about the world long before the overt appearance of traditional schizophrenic symptoms.

Among the earliest symptoms were disturbances in visual perception. For instance, one patient reported that even at an early stage, when he was thought by others to be reasonably normal, things were already changing:

> I was sitting listening to another person and suddenly the other person became smaller and then larger and then he seemed to get smaller again . . . . Then today with another person, I felt he was getting taller and taller. There is a brightness and clarity of outline of things around me. Last week I was with a girl and suddenly she seemed to get bigger and bigger, like a monster coming nearer and nearer. The situations become threatening and I shrink back and back.

Now this sounds almost like one who had taken a substantial dose of LSD. In fact, the "psychedelic" quality of the experiences of incipient schizophrenics has made many people wonder if the LSD "trip" might not be a drug model of schizophrenia. Here, it is worthwhile noticing how changes in perceptual filtering might result in bizarre changes in people's apparent size. The size of the image projected on the retina of our eyes, of course, varies with their distance from us, being much larger for objects which are closer and much smaller for far away objects. The brain has a talent for integrating the retinal images with other visual cues to let us know the real size of the object. In this way what we perceive is something or somebody of constant size, even though he moves closer to us or further away. A disruption of perceptual constancy might easily follow upon a weakening of the filtering and integrating powers of visual perception.

One of Chapman's patients explained quite clearly how his inability to sort out what is important from what is unimportant in things he perceives is sufficiently overwhelming that it forces his thoughts to grind to a halt. Such blockage is one of the most characteristic features of the schizophrenic thought disorder. As Chapman's patient puts it,

> it's like a temporary blackout—with my brain not working properly—like being in a vacuum. I just get cut off from outside things and go into another world. This happens when the tension starts to mount until it bursts in my brain. It has to do with what is going on around me—taking in too much of my surroundings—vital not to miss anything. I can't shut things out of my mind and everything closes in on me. It stops me thinking and then my goes blank and everything gets switched off. . . . I am observing everything around me.

Another of his patients remarked, "I can't control what's coming in and it stops me thinking with the mind a blank."

This same patient also described how his inability to hold off the bombardment of perceptual stimuli resulted in what sounds like the beginnings of catatonic paralysis of movement: "I take in too much so that I can't retain anything for any length of time—only a few seconds and I can't do simple habits like walking or cleaning my teeth . . . . When this starts I find myself having to use tremendous control to direct my feet and force myself round a corner as if I'm on a bicycle." The same perceptual flooding appeared to elicit in this patient typically schizophrenic feelings of disembodiment so that he was unable to experience the *self* of himself: "I find it difficult to cope with these situations, I get out of control and I can't differentiate myself from other people when this comes on."

Other patients also gave evidence of how their catatonic symptoms were actually at first a voluntary attempt to stabilize the world they were perceiving: "Everything is all right when I stop [moving]. If I move, everything I see keeps changing, everything I'm looking at gets broken up and I stop to put it together again." Or, as another patient observed, "When I start walking I get a fast series of pictures in front of me. Everything seems to change and revolve around me. Something goes wrong with my eyes and I've got to stop and stand still."

Of course it was not only perceptions which were affected in the early stages of schizophrenia. Just as they could not control their perceptions, so many of Chapman's patients reported that they could not control their thoughts, and again we are confronted with the problem of deciding whether perception regulates thought in schizophrenia or if it is the reverse. One of his patients said.

> I can't control my thoughts. I can't keep thoughts out. It comes on automatically. It happens at most peculiar times—not just when I'm talking but when I'm listening as well. I lose control in conversation, then I sweat and shake all over. . . . I can hear what they are saying all right, it's remembering what they have said in the next second that is difficult—it just goes out of my mind. I'm concentrating so much on little things I have difficulty in finding an answer at the time.

Here we can see how the intrusion of irrelevant thoughts and perceptions of what other people are doing or saying disrupted the thinking processes of Chapman's patient. It is almost as if sorting out the right elements in the environment upon which to focus one's attention and picking out from the treasury of one's recollections the appropriate reminiscence or concept are very closely related processes. Maybe the integration of sensory perception is regulated by the same mechanisms in the brain which control the filtering of perceptions of past thoughts and feelings.

Whether or not this is so, Chapman does attempt to describe how in most of his patients early disturbances in perception, and to a lesser extent cognition, gave rise to the whole panorama of schizophrenic manifestations.

> Most of the patients who experience this [perceptual] change reported that for a time everything around them looked fascinating, objects standing out vividly in contrast to the background. These initial changes were experienced as pleasant, and a number of patients at this stage went through a transient period of mild elation. Coincident with this alteration in perception, these patients appeared to regard everything with new significance, and there was a general tendency for their interests to be turned to ruminating about the world and life in general, and to religion, psychology, philosophy, art and literature.

Perhaps it is the flooding through the perceptual gates which results in the great vividness of the environment. And it is this vividness which makes the patient feel that everything that is happening is extraordinarily important. Of course such extremely significant occurrences taking place about them every day would seem to possess profound meaning. Here is the golden opportunity for the onset of delusional thinking about the world.

All of these unexplained perceptions cannot remain pleasant for long, and

> this early reaction changed to one of intense anxiety . . . that the patient could no longer see objects standing out clearly from the background and that instead they were

looking at many irrelevant aspects of the environment and were thus unable to perceive objects as meaningful wholes.

Chapman was also impressed at how so many secondary symptoms seemed to develop fairly directly out of the earlier changes in perception. We already mentioned how catatonic behavior was a device "to reduce quantitatively the intake of sensory stimulation from the environment at any particular time." Similarly Chapman thought that "social withdrawal was in part a voluntary activity carried out by the patient for his own protection." Moreover,

> as the various phenomena were continuously experienced, the patients gradually developed less rational and eventually floridly psychotic explanations to account for their experiences. Paranoid ideas and delusions of various kinds could be seen to develop in relation to the various categories of altered experience.

Thus Chapman feels that the symptoms of schizophrenic illness make their appearance in a sequential order, starting with disturbances of perception. Moreover, he has been impressed with how each disturbance develops out of preceding ones. Unfortunately, it is very difficult to learn just what is going on in the minds of schizophrenic patients at various stages of their illness. They are notoriously poor storytellers, and are likely to withhold what is most important. Moreover, in interviewing even normal subjects, the interviewer frequently finds what he is looking for by slanting his questions to elicit the information he is seeking.

Maybe Chapman was himself "misperceiving" the sequence of events in the unfolding of his patients' illness. Perhaps he was himself filtering out trends which he may not have wished to emphasize. Yet other authors have come to similar conclusions. Dr. Edward Ornitz reviews many published accounts by schizophrenic patients and their physicians detailing the stories of their disease, with a view to answering the question "Does disturbed [thinking] distort that which is perceived or does the disorder [in thinking] derive from a primary distortion of perception?" He finds evidence for an initial change of perceptual integration in a large number of case reports. A particularly convincing one was published by a patient herself in the *Journal of the Canadian Medical Association.*

She described a sequence of disturbances in her mental life which began with an "exaggerated state of awareness in which I lived, before, during, and after my acute illness." What is most notable about her account is her incisive analysis of how her illness developed:

Each of us is capable of coping with a large number of stimuli, invading our being through any one of the senses. We could hear every sound within earshot and see every object, line and color within the field of vision and so on. It is obvious that we would be incapable of carrying on any of our daily activities if even one-hundredth of all these available stimuli invaded us at once. So the mind must have a filter which functions without our conscious thought, sorting stimuli, and allowing only those which are relevant to the situation at hand to disturb consciousness. And this filter must be working at maximum efficiency at all times, particularly when we require a high degree of concentration. What had happened to me in Toronto was a breakdown in the filter, and a hodgepodge of unrelated stimuli were distracting me from things which should have had my undivided attention.

Thus it is fairly convincing that for *some* patients the onset of a schizophrenic illness is heralded by a disordered viewing of the external world, which then evolves into a tumultuous fragmentation of thinking and feeling.

Be Cautious

Whether events are ordered in this way for all patients is an open question. Morever, as far as we know, the disorders of perception, thinking and feeling in schizophrenia may be inextricably intertwined. Attempts to tease them apart may be fruitless because the disorders in these areas are held together by a common thread. Thus there may be some mechanism in the brain which pulls together stored memories and emotional states and tags them onto every incoming perception. If such a function were primarily at fault in schizophrenia, I suppose it could be called a "primary disturbance of perceptual integration." However, one would be hard put to prove it.

Despite all these caveats I think it is still worthwhile to propose a single, reasonably discrete failing in the mental processes of the schizophrenic. Certainly our hypothetical deficit fits in nicely with the neurophysiologic studies of how the antischizophrenic tranquilizers, the phenothiazine drugs, act in the brain. These drugs "tune down" the onslaught of the impinging world. By dampening the influence of perceptions on the patient's psychic life, the phenothiazines might be restoring the "filter" which seems to have been disarranged in the "perceiving" machinery of the schizophrenic mind.

9

Stimulants

Sigmund Freud may have done more for psychiatry than he ever thought possible, and in fact more than most professionals in psychiatry appreciate. Interestingly the one great deficiency of the psychoanalytic body of thought that Freud developed is that, both as a system or theory of mental functioning and as a therapeutic technique, it has little to offer for treating schizophrenia. Most psychiatrists agree that psychoanalytic theory has extraordinary value in helping to understand what makes people neurotic. In contrast, however, Freud's psychoanalytic formulations of schizophrenia have not really helped to illuminate the fundamental disturbances present in that disease. Predictably, psychoanalysis has not held up as a viable treatment for schizophrenia. Despite many heroic efforts by some of the leading psychoanalysts of this century, the best controlled research studies have all concluded that a simple prescription of chlorpromazine in adequate doses is far more useful for the schizophrenic patient than endless hours of love, trust and understanding on the part of the psychoanalytic therapist.

What then was Freud's real contribution to in understanding of schizophrenia? Many people are unaware of Freud's extensive career in medical research that preceded his discovery of psychoanalysis at the relatively late age of forty-one. Freud made some significant contributions to mapping the anatomy of the brain. In his capacity as a neurologist, he worked out mechanisms that determine the symptoms of aphasia, an inability to speak or express ideas which is most frequently manifested in people who have had strokes. In fact, it is something of a curious twist that, after devoting enormous effort to understanding why people cannot express themselves because of organic brain damage, that Freud should then make his greatest contribution in teaching people to express themselves via psychoanalysis, "the talking cure."

Freud's contribution to schizophrenia, as I see it, has to do with his introduction of cocaine to general medical awareness. For, in acting as the chief advocate for cocaine, Freud, more than any other single individual, was responsible for the extremely widespread use of cocaine throughout Europe and the United States in the latter part of the nineteenth century; for the subsequent epidemic of cocaine abuse; and for the phenomenon of "cocaine psychosis," which, along with amphetamine psychosis, may constitute the most meaningful drug model of schizophrenia.

About Cocaine

Although cocaine did not reach the attention of Europeans until the late nineteenth century, it had been enjoyed by Peruvian Indians, who chewed coca leaves for their stimulant effects, long before the white man reached America. A grave in Peru which dates from about A.D. 500 apparently contains one of the earliest records of the use of coca leaves. When Francisco Pizarro arrived in Peru in 1533, he discovered that the coca plant, *Erythroxylon coca* was already widely used. The coca leaf was an important part of the Inca culture and was even treated as money. Coca leaves were chewed much as Appalachian dwellers today chaw tobacco. Coca was treated with such respect and awe that it was incorporated into the Indian legends. It was said that the "children of the sun" (God's angels) had presented man with the coca leaf after the formation of the Inca empire to "satisfy the hungry, provide the weary and fainting with new vigor, and cause the unhappy to forget their miseries." This eloquent quotation tells us that the Peruvian Indians were already aware of the chief actions of cocaine: to suppress appetite, to enhance alertness, to promote muscular vigor, and to induce euphoria.

The Inca royalty attempted to reserve the use of coca to themselves. Its importance is evidenced by the fact that coca was a royal emblem; the Inca queen even called herself Momma Cuca, and the plant was used in religious ceremonies. The divine idols of the Incas were invariably depicted with one cheek stuffed with coca leaves.

Gradually the use of coca descended to the masses. Many writers have speculated that the psychotropic properties of coca deserve much of the credit for the incredible architectural feats of the Incas. For how else but by the energizing effects of coca could so many heavy loads of stones and wood have been carried across such high mountains? The ability of the drug to facilitate muscular activity even became a measure of time and distance in Peru. The "cocada" is defined as the distance, about three kilometers, which can be covered on a fairly flat surface under the influence of a standard dose of coca leaves; and for hilly terrain the cocada is only two kilometers.

Cocaine, which as we enter the decade of the 1970s is once again becoming a darling of the drug culture, was isolated from coca leaves by the German chemist Niemann in about 1859. Nothing much was done with it until the winter of 1883, when a Doctor von Aschen- brandt noticed that cocaine was useful in restoring the spirits and energy of German soldiers who had become fatigued after rigorous hiking exercises in the moun- tains.

Cocaine and Sigmund Freud

Sigmund Freud, then working as a neuropathologist in a Viennese hospital, was quick to recognize that this sort of effect might be uniquely valuable in psychiatry. For, as he puts it himself, "psychiatry is rich in drugs that can subdue overstimulated nervous activity, but deficient in agents that can heighten the performance of the depressed nervous system."

Even before doing any experiments with the drug— in fact before he had obtained a supply of it—Freud was enormously enthusiastic and sure that he was onto a miracle drug. He viewed this as an opportunity to "make" his career, obtain a promotion, more money, and thus finally be in a position to marry his fiancée, to whom he had been engaged by this time for over two years. His letters to her convey his enthusiasm:

I have been reading about cocaine, the essential constituent of coca leaves which some Indian tribes chewed to enable them to resist privations and hardships. A German has been employing it with soldiers and has in fact reported that it increases their energy and capacity to endure. I am procuring some myself and will try it with cases of heart disease and also of nervous exhaustion, particularly in the miserable condition after withdrawal of morphine. Perhaps others are working at it; perhaps nothing will come of it. But I shall certainly try it, and you know that when one perseveres, sooner or later one succeeds. We do not need more than one such lucky hit to be able to think of setting up house.

As soon as he was able to purchase cocaine from the Merck Drug Company, he swallowed some of it himself. He quickly discovered the central stimulant actions of cocaine, which are very much like those of amphetamine. It produced in him a moderate euphoria, made feel more alert, resistant to fatigue, and devoid of appetite. Soon he was taking cocaine regularly, recommending it to everyone he knew, and trying it out in almost every conceivable medical condition. He conveyed this exuberance in his letters to his fiancée, "I take . . . it regularly against depression and against indigestion and with the most brilliant success. I hope I will be able to abolish the most intractable vomiting, even when this is due to severe pain."

One of the features which cocaine and amphetamines seem to share is the ability to stimulate sexual appetite in some people, just as it abolishes the appetite for food and makes the user feel boundlessly energetic. Sigmund Freud may have been one such individual, as he wrote to his Martha, "woe to you my princess when I come. I will kiss you quite red and feed you until you are plump. And if you are forward, you shall see who is the stronger, a gentle little girl who doesn't eat enough or a *big wild man who has cocaine in his body.*"

As with amphetamines, cocaine provokes a sense of well-being which can move some users to a state of veritable ecstasy. Freud said "I am just now busy collecting the literature for a song of praise to this magical substance." The "song of praise" was to be Freud's scientific description of cocaine and its effects in himself and in a number of patients, a publication which literally "turned on" European medicine to the possibilities of this remarkable drug.

Freud summarized his major findings in this way:

Cocaine brings about an exhilaration and lasting euphoria which in no way differs from the normal euphoria of the healthy person . . . you perceive an increase of self-control and possess more vitality and capacity for work . . . in other words, you are simply normal, and it is soon hard to believe that you are under the influence of any drug . . . long intensive mental or physical work is performed without any fatigue . . . this result is enjoyed without any of the unpleasant aftereffects that follow exhilaration brought about by alcohol.

Though Freud observed that cocaine abolished his appetite, it never occurred to him that the drug might be used for weight reduction. Probably this is simply because, in the late nineteenth century Austria, being plump was the essence of fashionable attractiveness. Skinny women either were too poor to eat well or were suspected of being tuberculous.

According to today's tradition of psychiatric pigeon-holing, we would consider Sigmund Freud to have been chronically depressed at a neurotic level. By neurotic depression, I mean to contrast his condition with severe or "psychotic" depression, in which the afflicted individuals are unable to work, sleep, and often eat. Though Freud's spirits were often low, he was a highly effective worker. What excited him most about cocaine was its ability to relieve his feelings of depression. Probably the apparent "antidepressant" actions of cocaine, like those of amphetamine, spring from the ability of the drug to provoke euphoria, an artificial feeling of enhanced well-being. One is euphoric if he feels happier than we physicians judge to be his just desert.

Nowadays we know that cocaine as well as amphetamine is a tremendously addicting drug. An individual taking cocaine a few times soon finds it is necessary to escalate the dose to produce the same effect which was originally elicited by a small amount of the drug. This escalation often assumes mammoth proportions, with addicts consuming 100 times as much drug as they had first used. Along with the "tolerance" to massive amounts of the drug, addiction to cocaine brings with it a compulsive desire to take cocaine; in fact it is probably the compulsive drug-seeking behavior which is far more crucial to the concept of "addiction" than any other aspect of drug use, whether it be tolerance or the presence of withdrawal symptoms. This all-consuming craving for the drug occurs with all drug addictions including amphetamines, heroin, barbiturates, alcohol, and nicotine, as well as cocaine.

Curiously, with cocaine and amphetamine only some people are susceptible to addiction. Sigmund Freud was not one of those unlucky ones. Accordingly, since most of his research with cocaine was conducted upon himself, he concluded and published in his classic paper on cocaine the notion that cocaine was not at all addicting, "absolutely no craving for the further use of cocaine appears after the first, or even repeated, taking of the drug."

Because Freud thought that cocaine was not addict-

ing, he recommended it for use in withdrawing morphine addicts from their addiction. His first patient was
a physician friend of his who had become addicted to
morphine after using the drug to treat the excruciating
pain of a severed thumb. After taking cocaine, the friend
was able to dispense with morphine. But within a period
of a few months he had become a severe cocaine
addict, perhaps the first in Europe, and gradually increased his dose to more than 100 times what he had
first taken. His friend's addiction was not apparent until
after Freud had already published his essay on cocaine.
Thus Freud, to his later regret, waxed eloquent in his
publication about the remarkable nature of cocaine, the
only psychotropic drug to be *totally free* of addictive
potential.

Soon after Freud's publication doctors throughout
Europe were prescribing cocaine for all sorts of conditions, especially for people who like Freud were neurotically depressed, chronically fatigued, and unhappy
about life in general. Unfortunately, such individuals are
especially prone to becoming addicted to almost any
drug. Soon in all countries of Europe there were large
numbers of cocaine addicts in all walks of life. Not only
were patients put on the drug by their physicians, but,
as has taken place in modern times, there soon developed a vigorous black market in the drug, which was
sought out solely as a pleasure-producing agent.

The situation at the turn of the century was aptly
described by the pharmacologist Lewis Lewin,

> [A]lready in 1901 there were many cocainistic men and
> women in England, doctors, politicians, and writers. At
> present the situation is evidently much worse, although
> morphinism has not been dethroned. In Germany, mainly in
> the large towns, there are many cocainists in every profes-

sion, down to prostitutes and their protectors. In certain bars and restaurants, in the street, etc., cocaine is clandestinely sold, very frequently stolen or adulterated into merchandise for which huge prices, up to 30 marks, are asked and paid. In Berlin there are cocaine dens, both disreputable and dirty and also fashionable and up-to-date establishments. One of these was raided by the police at the beginning of the present year. About 100 habitués, men and women from all classes of society, even university and literary men, had gathered there to lead for a few hours an existence of unreality. They spent whole days without taking food . . . they gave all that they possessed, even indispensable articles of clothing, in order to indulge their mad craving. The most fantastic description of the night side of human life, the sketch of Hogarth representing a party of punch drinkers and like works which show the vileness of the human individual fallen to a level below that of the beasts, cannot equal in horror the picture of degradation presented by such an assembly in the throes of cocaine.

Thus Freud, about ten years before he was to revolutionize psychiatry by his discovery of psychoanalysis, sparked a drug abuse epidemic in Europe which may well rival the American bout with drugs of abuse in the 1960s. Indeed, within a few years after cocaine was introduced into European medicine, it was labeled by the eminent German physician Erlenmeyer as "the third scourge of humanity," the other two being alcohol and morphine addiction. For years afterwards, Sigmund Freud alternately berated himself for his premature enthusiastic disclosure of cocaine and rationalized his actions by blaming others.

Cocaine Craziness

What benefit can so seemingly heinous drug as cocaine bring to us in our attempt to understand the brain dysfunction in schizophrenia? And if Freud's contribution to the cocaine subject was merely to provoke widespread abuse of the drug, how can his seemingly misjudgment have had anything to offer psychiatry? Ironically, Freud's contribution is specifically his lack of scientific discretion. For without his premature conclusions there would have been no cocaine epidemic, no cocaine addicts, and thus no discovery of a major side affect of cocaine addiction—and the one of greatest interest to us—namely, cocaine psychosis.

Cocaine psychosis, which occurs quite frequently in cocaine addicts, is virtually indistinguishable from acute paranoid schizophrenia. Many patients with cocaine psychosis were misdiagnosed as paranoid schizophrenics until the history of drug use was apparent. The sequence of events is usually as follows. After having ingested cocaine for a period of weeks in massive doses, the addict will gradually become suspicious. Soon he will feel that the police, his friends, or someone from outer space is after him. In an effort to defend himself from his persecutors, the cocaine psychotic may become dangerously violent. He will invariably arm himself, often with a gun, and will not hesitate to kill whoever he views as a threat. Along with these delusions of persecution, the cocaine psychotic often hears voices. Besides such auditory hallucinations, he may have tactile hallucinations, feeling that small animals— worms, ants, lice—are creeping beneath his skin. Often he imagines that enemies have implanted cocaine crystals under his skin. The reality of these hallucinations may be so great that the addict will pierce his skin with needles to try to pick out the foreign bodies.

Some psychiatrists have argued that cocaine psychosis should never be mistaken for schizophrenia, because the individual under the influence of cocaine does not display the characteristic thought disorder of schizophrenics and does not have the typically schizophrenic disturbance of feeling responses to the environment. However, other psychiatrists question that there are any differences of a major sort between the symptoms of cocaine psychosis and those of paranoid schizophrenia. They simply point out that the large number of cocaine psychotics upon whom the label of schizophrenia was affixed by reputable psychiatrists bespeaks a fundamental similarity between the entities.

All of this suggests that cocaine psychosis might be a useful drug model for schizophrenia. And, as we discussed before in relationship to the psychedelic drugs, drug models may provide a powerful means for discovering the fundamental brain disturbances in schizophrenia. During the late nineteenth and twentieth century when cocaine addiction and psychosis were prevalent in Europe, psychiatrists did not write much about drug models of schizophrenia and rarely, if ever, mentioned cocaine as a "model schizophrenia." Probably the reason was that schizophrenia as a diagnostic entity was not well established until Bleuler's famous monograph of 1911, and even after that it took some time for the concept of schizophrenia to percolate throughout the intellectual framework of conventional psychiatry.

Amphetamine

The effects of cocaine are mimicked almost perfectly by amphetamine, known to many today as "speed." As already mentioned, amphetamine and cocaine share the ability to produce euphoria and alertness, to increase muscular energy, to suppress appetite, and even to stimulate sexual desire. And they also share the ability to produce psychoses which are very much like paranoid schizophrenia. Amphetamine psychosis, being a creature of the mid-twentieth-century age of vigorous psychiatric research, has been studied much more closely than cocaine psychosis. Thus we would do well to shift our attention now to the amphetamines.

Chemically, amphetamine and cocaine are very different; however, in terms of their psychotropic properties, the two drugs are quite similar, if not identical. Yet when amphetamine was introduced into clinical medicine in the 1930s no one noticed its similarity to cocaine. It took a while for the medical profession to "discover" the various properties of amphetamine— properties which, for all practical purposes, were the same as those of cocaine. This similarity holds true as well for the abuse potential of both drugs. Amphetamine addiction is every bit as overwhelming an experience as is cocaine addiction. It has taken us almost forty years since the introduction of amphetamine to recognize the simple fact of its abuse potential—something which an astute pharmacologist should have been able to proclaim in 1938 or earlier.

Perhaps one reason the medical profession has been so tardy in recognizing the various psychotropic properties of the amphetamines is that amphetamine came into the purview of organized medicine by a completely different route then did cocaine. Freud introduced cocaine to Europe specifically as a central stimulant, a euphoria-producing agent. By contrast, amphetamine came to us as a new medication for the relief of bronchial asthma.

The Speed Story

It had been known for many years that one of the most effective treatments for asthma is epinephrine, or adrenalin, the hormone secreted by the medullary part of the adrenal gland. Indeed, it is quite likely that epinephrine secretion from the adrenal gland normally plays a prominent role in regulating the diameter of the bronchi and hence is a normal circulating "antiasthmatic." Unfortunately, epinephrine is relatively unstable as a chemical and cannot be taken by mouth. The Chinese-American pharmacologist Dr. K. K. Chen had been systematically investigating the ancient Chinese drug codification and noticed repeated mention of a desert plant *ma huang* as a treatment for asthma. The botanical name for the *ma huang* plant is *Ephedra vulgaris*. Chen tried out a chemical extracted from the plant, which was called ephedrine, in asthmatic patients. Ephedrine turned out to be extraordinarily successful in the treatment of asthma, especially since it could be taken by mouth.

Fairly soon it became obvious that the plant supplies from which ephedrine was obtained might soon be exhausted. At this point, Gordon Alles, a chemist who had been working in the clinical laboratories of an allergist attempting to make a series of purified proteins for use in allergy testing, became interested in the possibility of developing a synthetic substitute for ephedrine. Amphetamine was the most successful of the series of chemicals he made.

Like many other chemicals, amphetamine can exist in two mirrorlike forms because its structure is inherently asymmetric. The two forms of amphetamine are identical in every way except that they are literally mirror images of each other. The way in which chemists can tell the difference between the two is to shine a beam of polarized light at them. One form rotates light to the right—*dextro* in Greek—while the other rotates it to the left—*levo*. Only after he has synthesized the amphetamine as a mixture of both forms was Alles able to separate dextroamphetamine from levoamphetamine.

As was his wont, Alles immediately tried the two drugs out on himself. It was quite evident to him that dextroamphetamine, the form that rotates light to the right, was more active. It was at least four to five times as potent a central stimulate as the levo form of the drug. Accordingly, though the Smith, Kline, and French drug company provided levoamphetamine with the brand name Levedrine at the same time that it was christening dextroamphetamine as Dexedrine, Levedrine has been left relatively untouched by the medical profession over the years, and has been treated largely as a waste by-product in the manufacture of dextroamphetamine.

What brought Alles his greatest commercial success was his ability to prepare amphetamine in a form which was volatile, which means that it could be formed readily into vapors and used as an inhaler. The Smith, Kline, and French Company also developed this into an immensely successful marketing enterprise of "benzedrine" (the trade name for amphetamine) inhalers.

Like Freud, Gordon Alles experimented extensively upon himself and in this way very quickly was able to recognize the various psychotropic activities of amphetamine. He noted that the drug made him feel euphoric, enhanced his abilities to focus on intellectual work, and prevented fatigue. Somewhat later he recognized the appetite suppressing activities of the drug. Also, like

Freud, he had not the faintest intimation that amphetamine could possibly be addicting. All of organized medicine and the Food and Drug Administration seemed to have little more insight into the abuse potential than did Alles himself. For the drug was approved by the FDA for prescription as a tool to capture "a sense of increased energy or capacity for work, or a feeling of exhilaration." Thus the Food and Drug Administration in the morally repressive, Calvinistic United States was clearly authorizing the prescription of a drug for work purposes, something to "feel good"—almost, perhaps, like advocating marijuana.

What Amphetamine May Be Good For

Again, as with cocaine, amphetamine was widely prescribed as an antidepressant, especially for people with mild neurotic depression. Nowadays the medical profession recognizes, at least in theory, that the use of amphetamine for the treatment of depression is rather questionable, because mildly neurotically depressed people are those who are most liable to become abusers of the drugs. Surprisingly, however, some amphetamine derivatives, especially the drug methylphenidate (Ritalin), are still widely advertised in medical journals as agents to relieve mild depression.

In the late 1930s the commercial potential of amphetamine's capacity to suppress appetite became evident, a property which had escaped the adherents of cocaine fifty years earlier. The vast numbers of American housewives who were obese, mildly plump, or who simply thought that they would be more beautiful if skinnier, became legitimate hunting grounds for the ingenuity of the public relations departments of the drug companies.

Chemists worked furiously, grinding out different analogues of amphetamine to the patent which the Smith, Kline, and French Company held on amphetamine itself. It was found that certain of these amphetamine derivatives tended to have somewhat more potency in suppressing appetite than in causing central stimulation. These drugs, in theory, should provoke less insomnia and be less subject to abuse. Among these specialized "diet pills" are such well known drugs as phenmetrazine (Preludin), diethylpropion (Tenuate), and phendimetrazine (Plegine). Unfortunately, while in animals there may be some separation of the central stimulant and appetite-suppressing activities, in man and woman the difference between these effects of these drugs is not pronounced. In fact, in Sweden during the tremendous amphetamine abuse epidemic of the 1950s, when the government clamped down on the distribution of amphetamine itself, there emerged rapidly an even more widespread epidemic of Preludin abuse.

Other amphetamine analogues were synthesized in an effort to eliminate the appetite-suppressing activity and to retain exclusively central stimulant properties. The best known of these agents is methylphenidate, whose brand name is Ritalin. Ritalin is currently widely prescribed for the relief of minor depression, specifically because the drug ought not to interfere with the user's appetite. As best I can gather, this is indeed a valid claim. Ritalin users do not complain much about a lack of interest in food. Whether or not the drug is really useful in relieving depression is more questionable.

One completely legitimate medical use is the treatment of narcolepsy. Narcolepsy is a rare condition in which people tend to fall asleep inexplicably and while engaged in some activity which should have kept them alert. In my lectures to students I find the most apt description is something like this: "If you people in the audience should be falling asleep now, that is perfectly normal. But if I should fall asleep, that would be narcolepsy." Narcolepsy was the first medical condition in which amphetamine was employed, and it continues to be the least controversial aspect of the use of the drug. The rationale is straightforward and the drug is generally quite effective. However, narcoleptics often do become tolerant to the effects of amphetamine and are required to greatly increase the doses. Some of them have developed amphetamine psychosis as a result.

Hyperactive Kids, a Special Case

Another medical use for which amphetamine is certainly quite justified is the hyperactive syndrome in children. This condition is also called "minimal brain dysfunction," although no one has been able to demonstrate rigorously the presence of abnormal brain functioning in these children. These hyperactive children usually have normal intelligence. However, their parents describe a peculiar situation in which, since earliest babyhood, they were simply quite "hyperactive." "Johnny never sat still in his life. Even when he was two years old, if we took our eyes off him for one minute he would be climbing on top of the bookcase in the other end of the house." In school such children literally drive their teachers to distraction. Teachers are especially frustrated, because children with the hyperactive syndrome are not malicious and hence the teacher feels guilty for repeatedly punishing them. However, they are unable to stay in one place, constantly irritate the other children, and disrupt all class proceedings.

As one might expect, since they are never in one place, it is quite difficult for these children to maintain an adequate focus of attention on their school work. Therefore, although they are of normal intelligence, children with the hyperactive syndrome do quite poorly in their school work.

These children respond dramatically to the administration of amphetamines. Within a few hours after the children have ingested the first pill, their mothers will inform the physician that the child has been transformed into a virtual angel. Under the influence of amphetamines, these children become placid and hyperconscientious. They are rapidly moved to tears when rebuked. Fortunately, rebuke is no longer necessary. Several investigators have been able to demonstrate a definite increase in the I.Q. scores of these children when placed on amphetamines. All of this is especially remarkable in light of the fact that amphetamines make adults hyperexcited, talkative, and less able to sit still than previously.

How does one account for this paradoxical calming effect of amphetamines in the hyperactive children? Scientists are not at all sure just how to explain the differential responses to amphetamines of hyperactive children and adults. The situation is especially perplexing because normal children respond to amphetamines much like adults, becoming exceedingly jittery. Conceivably, what is going on is something like the following: Maybe amphetamines are not "calming" the hyperactive children in the sense of a sedative drug. Rather, just as in adults, amphetamine enhances the alertness of the hyperactive children. Perhaps their difficulty had been that they were unable to concentrate on their school work, to focus their attention on any one subject for a prolonged period of time. By making them more alert, amphetamine enables them to focus their concentration. It prolongs their attention span, and thus seems to the observer to be quieting them down.

Still, there are other paradoxical aspects of the influence of these drugs upon hyperactive children. While 10 milligrams of dextroamphetamine would be enough to render a 150-pound man exceedingly alert, jittery, and insomniac, hyperactive children weighing only one-third as much tolerate doses of dextroamphetamine of up to 40 milligrams per day without any apparent adverse effects. There may be a slight loss of appetite and minor insomnia in some of them, but many have no insomnia or appetite suppression whatsoever.

How many children suffer from the hyperactive syndrome? It is quite difficult to make a meaningful estimate. The condition is not readily diagnosed in a rigorous fashion. One cannot take a throat culture as one does to diagnose a strep throat. Instead, one must rely on a constellation of symptoms of abnormal behavior. And usually the clincher to the diagnosis is the patient's response to amphetamine administration. Enormous numbers of children misbehave in school. Probably only a minority of these suffer from the classic hyperactive syndrome. The simplest approach is to try a test dose of amphetamine. If the child becomes worse than he was before, nervous and unable to sleep, then he probably does not possess the condition, whereas, if his symptoms improve, this establishes a diagnosis. On the basis of attempts to diagnose children in this way, there have been estimates that perhaps as many as five to fifteen percent of American schoolchilren suffer from the hyperactive syndrome.

Because hyperactivity is a vaguely defined condition and because the drug used to treat it is one which is well known to be potentially addictive, opponents of this treatment say that it represents a means by which organized medicine and teachers can control the minds of children. The specter of *1984* has been raised. However, these concerns are pretty much unjustified. The hyperactive syndrome tends to disappear by puberty. And there is no evidence whatsoever that these children manifest even the slightest tendency to become addicted to the drug or abuse it in any way. If anything, there is evidence that, if untreated, children with the hyperactive syndrome are likely to turn to antisocial behavior as adolescents and adults. Thus, these children, if not regulated by amphetamines, go through school for years and years being labeled as "bad ones." Not surprisingly, they adopt for themselves the image foisted upon them by their teachers and parents. Naturally they will then have a much greater chance than the average child of becoming juvenile delinquents. With amphetamine treatment, there is strong evidence that they function as normal children and have little difficulty in functioning normally in society once they reach adolescence and adulthood.

When Amphetamine Is Bad, It Is Very Bad

It should not be too surprising that this drug which makes one feel very very good has an enormous abuse potential. The first amphetamine addicts were reported in the late 1930s. These individuals would ingest the entire contents of a benzedrine (the mixture of dextro- and levoamphetamine) inhaler in a single dose. Each inhaler contained 250 milligrams of the drug or about twenty-five times the dose which would suffice to stimulate a normal adult.

In 1938 several cases were reported of individuals who developed a paranoid psychosis from the chronic use of massive doses of amphetamines via the inhalers. Also about that time some chronic abuse of amphetamine pills began in the United States.

It is said that some students of the University of Minnesota first recognized the value of amphetamine pills for keeping themselves awake throughout several consecutive nights in order to study for final exams. This fad caught on with remarkable speed. Even today amphetamines are widely used by college students to assist in "burning the midnight oil" at exam time. In the late 1930s the popular press helped in spreading this information and sensationalizing the dangers but at the same time making the drug seem quite fascinating, thus presumably contributing to further abuse. References to amphetamines in the popular press included "pep pills," "superman pills," and "brain pills."

After students, the next major class of American heavy abusers of amphetamines were the coast-to-coast truck drivers, who consumed the drug to facilitate all-night drives. There have been tragic motorcar and truck accidents resulting from truck driving while under the influence of so large a dose of amphetamine that the driver was fully psychotic.

Amphetamine abuse gained an international flavor in World War II. The Germans deserve the credit for the development of methamphetamine, which differs from amphetamine itself only in the addition of carbon and three hydrogens to the molecule. Although the matter is not altogether clear, it seems that methamphetamine produces somewhat more euphoria than amphetamine itself; hence, it is the true darling of the drug set. The term "speed," strictly defined (if that is possible in the drug culture), refers specifically to methamphetamine, although many people use the term when they are talking about amphetamines in general.

The German armed forces used methamphetamine to keep their pilots alert during all-night air raids over England. The British armed forces readily dispensed amphetamine tablets to all their soldiers. Interestingly, scientific and medical consultants to the American army vigorously debated whether amphetamine ought to be administered to American troops. Chauncey Leake, an American pharmacologist, who himself authored a book on the amphetamines about fifteen years ago, strongly advocated the use of amphetamine by American troops. He was overruled by Dr. Andrew Ivy, a prominent American physiologist, who argued that amphetamines might be too toxic for this purpose. However, since all our Allies were using amphetamines, the drugs were simply dispensed to American soldiers by British army physicians.

Lester Grinspoon, in surveying the history of amphetamine abuse, concluded that the amount of benzedrine supplied to U.S. servicemen by the British in World War II was about 80,000,000 tablets. Perhaps another eighty to 100 million tablets were obtained one way or another through the U.S. army medics. He concludes that at an absolute minimum ten percent of American fighting men must have used amphetamines during World War II; and, if so, then more than 1.5 million of them returned to this country with some first-hand knowledge of the effects of the drug.

Meanwhile, during World War II, the United States armed forces were conducting research to resolve the question of whether amphetamines would be useful for our soldiers. One such purportedly scientific study cast as much light upon the activities and techniques for training soldiers as it does on the effects of amphetamines:

> 100 marines were kept active continuously for 60 hours in range firing, a 25-mile forced march, a field problem, calisthenics, close-ordered drill games, fatigue detail, and bivouac alerts. Fifty men received seven 10 milligram tablets of benzedrine at six hour intervals following the first day's activity. Meanwhile the other fifty were given placebo (milk sugar) tablets. None knew what he was receiving. Participating officers concluded that the benzedrine definitely "pepped up" the subjects, improved their morale, reduced sleepiness and increased confidence in shooting ability . . . it was observed that men receiving benzedrine tended to lead the march, tolerate their sore feet and blisters more cheerfully, and remain wide awake during "breaks," whereas members of the control group had been shaken to keep them from sleeping.

Amphetamines did indeed catch on among the American soldiers, as attested to by the report in 1947 that at least twenty-five percent of prisoners in an army stockade were heavy and chronic users of amphetamines.

The Japanese obtained large quantities of methamphetamine from their German allies. In contrast to the Germans, however, they used them more for civilians than for soldiers. Japanese munitions factory workers used methamphetamine almost compulsively in order to keep up their spirit and efficiency, and Japanese drug companies therefore built up enormous stocks of them. To encourage the comsumption of amphetamines, the Japanese brand name was identical with their proposed function. Amphetamine was dubbed "wakeamine."

With the war's end, Japanese drug companies endeavored to clean out their huge stock piles by advertising "amphetamine for elimination of drowsiness and repletion of the spirit." This ad campaign seems to have appealed to many young Japanese who had suffered from frustration and loss of self-confidence during the profound demoralization which swept their country after the war. There soon followed the world's first true amphetamine epidemic. By May 1954 it was estimated that one percent of the entire population of the city of Kurume in Japan was addicted. Moreover, about five percent of all Japanese between the ages of sixteen and twenty-five were addicts to the drug. Naturally, with so many amphetamine addicts, one should not be surprised that the common sequelae of addiction should result—amphetamine psychosis with all its paranoid features and their fatal outcome. During May and June 1954, out of sixty murder cases in Japan, thirty-one of the murderers had some connection with amphetamine use. Only by extraordinarily strict regulations were the Japanese able to quell the epidemic. The manufacture of amphetamines was strictly regulated and the government imposed six-month jail sentences for simple illegal possession of the drug. In about three years, the epidemic seems to have withered away.

Widespread use of amphetamines appeared next in Sweden. The pattern here was particularly interesting, inasmuch as governmental suppression of amphetamine seems to have sparked the epidemic to its greatest ferocity. Amphetamine itself had been labeled as a narcotic in Sweden since the mid-1940s. However, there was a gradually increasing abuse of amphetamine pills obtained illegally by prescription. To stem the illegal use of amphetamines, the government placed a total ban on the prescription of these drugs. However, they did not include the supposedly nonabusable amphetamine analogues which were used for weight reduction, especially Preludin. Soon every legal and illegal source of Preludin was being tapped to supply a demand far greater than that which had existed for amphetamine itself. Preludin was used orally and, to a limited extent, injected intravenously.

Living—Or Dying—With Speed

Amphetamine abuse in its most exuberant and heinous enormity came to the United States in the late 1960s, taking the form of a speed epidemic caused by the systematic intravenous dosing of amphetamines. It started with the hippies in San Francisco. To heighten the intensity of the psychedelic experience, some bold ones added methamphetamine to preparations of LSD. It was said that LSD spiked with methamphetamine gave a keener and more euphoric experience than LSD itself. Methamphetamine was the favorite amphetamine, according to the folklore of the drug set, because it produced more euphoria than others. Also, it was the only amphetamine widely available from manufacturers in a liquid form suitable for intravenous injection. In any event, from the enclaves of the hippies there emerged the speed freak. He was not able to tolerate the overwhelming self-revelation induced by LSD and preferred instead to be high, pure and simple, with speed.

Dr. John Kramer has traced the California epidemic of the intravenous use of amphetamine in the 1960s. He feels that it all began in 1960–1961 when some physicians in San Francisco began prescribing large amounts of injectable methamphetamine to patients who identified themselves as heroin addicts. Since it is doubtful that heroin addicts would be at all interested in amphetamine, the physicians were presumably duped. In any event, these doctors erroneously reasoned, much like Sigmund Freud eighty years before, that amphetamines would help the opiate addict resist heroin. As the authorities came to recognize the abuse potential of injectable methamphetamine, it was rapidly removed from pharmacies. However, the appetite of users had been whetted. They soon discovered that they could purchase crystalline methamphetamine in large quantities from manufacturers simply by representing themselves as pharmacological researchers. And after that source dried up because of federal regulation, underground chemists began the manufacture of methamphetamine for the illicit market which, by the late 1960s, represented the major source.

The typical pattern for intravenous speed use is to inject it about every two hours around the clock for three to six days, during which time the user remains continuously awake, excited, and somewhat paranoid. Sometimes these "runs" last as long as twelve days, after which the addict "crashes." Crashing is a state in which the user is so exhausted, disorganized, and confused that he ceases using the drug and goes to sleep. Sleep is profound and so deep that the user can rarely be awakened. After a three-day run the user may sleep for eighteen hours; while after longer runs, some patients stay unconscious for four or five days. Once awake, the amphetamine addict is ravenously hungry, no longer agitated or paranoid, but still fatigued. He eats and eats and continues to rest until, after a vacation of three to four days, he is ready to start again on another run.

What is the attraction of a drug which so disorganizes the user and which provokes in almost every addict at one time or another a terrifying paranoid psychosis? The addicts seem most to seek the sensation obtained immediately following intravenous injection. There is a sudden, generalized, overwhelming feeling of pleasure, referred to as a "rush" or "flash." Many users compare it to a whole body orgasm, and in this way it resembles the flash following intravenous injection of heroin. The one major difference between amphetamine and heroin self-administration is that the amphetamine user feels an abrupt awakening sensation shortly after administering the drug, while the heroin user becomes drowsy.

While we have spoken of the influence of orally administered amphetamine as being "euphoric," this is too pallid a description for the experience which follows intravenous injection. The user becomes intensely fascinated with every aspect of his body and the world about him in an ineffable fashion.

Most amphetamine addicts become totally engrossed in sexual desire, although a limited number lose interest. For the speed freak sexual intercourse is a glorious enterprise. Ejaculation is delayed in the male as is orgasm in the female. Thus partners will carry on intercourse continuously as long as twelve hours or more, and, when orgasm finally occurs, it is far more powerful and pleasurable then anything ever experienced without the drug. Gösta Rylander, a Swedish physician, has concluded that amphetamine must be the most powerful aphrodisiac known. He quoted a patient who said that an injection of amphetamine "goes straight from the head to the scrotum . . . this wonderful drug is a fucking pump . . . I always need a couple of girls at the same time."

Gail Sheehy describes how some users feel about amphetamine,

> the magic vitamin. Ups, speed, amphetamine. It is all the same. What makes everyone fall in love with amphetamine is the magic of feeling like the beautiful, confident, convivial person we all want to be all the time. It was good when he slipped the needle in for her. RUSH from vein to brain in less than one second. Her old self-hating self died. She was reborn. He [her boyfriend who has just turned her on to amphetamines] renamed her Joy. Now they never have to go out for anything . . . for the Superior Man [the self-image of the amphetamine addict], and his Joy, stay in as a groove. It is retirement at 23.

One unique feature of amphetamine addicts is the compulsive stereotyped behavior they display. Hour after hour apparently without fatigue or boredom, they will continue to repeat the same activity. One woman sorted out her handbag over and over for hours on end. Mechanically inclined individuals have been known to spend many hours trying to dismantle and repair gadgets which were in perfect order. One patient "collected a dozen radios which he took apart in order to build a new one. It did not matter to him that he did not succeed. Another member of the group who paid him a visit at that time said, 'he cheerfully kept himself busy and nothing could divert him from this foolish task.' " This strange stereotyped compulsive behavior is often accompanied by teeth gritting and strange facial grimaces. Interestingly, with relatively high doses of amphetamines, animals display extremely similar patterns of behavior. Were we able to determine experimentally exactly what changes in the brain mediate these behaviors in animals, we would accordingly have some insight into these aspects of amphetamine action in man.

The slogan "speed kills" is familiar to anyone who has read much about the drug culture in America. Amphetamine itself does not directly kill the user. In fact, surveys of the most heavy users of intravenous amphetamine in California (individuals who have self-injected up to 1000 or more milligrams per day) have failed to reveal more than a few cases of death from overdose. What the slogan refers to is the propensity of individuals, while in a paranoid psychotic state under the influence of the drug, to lash out at their "tormenters" with fatal consequences. As mentioned earlier, in Japan at one point fully half of the murderers arrested within a two-month period were heavy amphetamine users.

In the United States, Everett Ellinwood, a psychiatrist at Duke University, has catalogued the histories of thirteen homicides committed under the influence of amphetamine. These constitute a grim testimony to the consequences of the use of this drug. One of Dr. Ellinwood's cases was

> a twenty-seven-year-old truck driver who shot his boss in the back of the head because he thought the boss was trying to release poison gas into the back seat of the car in which he was riding. "I thought they had gassed me. My boss kept reaching down beside him and pulling on something. I rolled down the window to let the gas out. I got nauseated and passed out due to the gas; I then got up on my elbow and shot my boss, who was driving."

Over the previous twenty hours, in order to make a non-stop 1,600 mile trip, the patient had ingested 180 milligrams of amphetamine and had not slept for 48 hours. . . . Six to eight hours before the murder he had become increasingly suspicious that someone had planted drugs on his truck . . . he called a highway patrolman, related his suspicions in a bizarre manner and was taken to the local jail for safe keeping, where he hallucinated, "then there were muffled voices in the next room and they tried to gas me. I could hear the hissing. I got down and looked under the door; I saw feet there."

Another patient of Dr. Ellinwood's was a woman who had received amphetamines to help her lose weight.

However she soon discovered that they relieved her loneliness and depression; gradually over a period of 18 months, she increased the dose to 400 to 600 mg per day. She hallucinated and became suspicious, "even the people who were helping me were against me." She bought a pistol to protect herself and her children at night. Then during an argument with her boyfriend, she pulled a pistol out of her waistband, stuck it in his stomach and calmly fired. When the victim got out of the car, she followed him and stated "you wanted to die; I showed you." She then shot him twice more and turned to a bystander, saying "Turn him over and take a picture of his pretty face."

10

Amphetamine Psychosis: A Clue to Mechanisms of Madness?

The aspect of amphetamine use which may hold the greatest value in our search for fundamental disturbances in schizophrenia is amphetamine psychosis. There are at least two types of psychotic reactions which can follow amphetamine use, only one of which is of interest to us. Like most other drugs, amphetamine can cause a toxic psychosis in which the patient is delirious, confused, and does not know what time it is, where he is, or who he is. This is very much like the psychoses which occur in the presence of a high fever, with vitamin deficiency, or with any of a number of drugs. For instance, delirium tremens is a condition in which alcoholics, usually soon after terminating a prolonged binge, become psychotic. They are confused, don't know who they are, where they are, or what time of day it is. They experience vivid and terrifying visual hallucinations, such as seeing pink elephants on the walls coming after them. During the "toxic" psychosis with amphetamine there also are visual hallucinations.

The toxic psychosis, however, tells us nothing about schizophrenia. As we discussed previously in relationship to the psychedelic drugs, for a model psychosis to have relevance for schizophrenia it should occur in a setting of clear consciousness in which the patient is alert and aware of who he is, where he is, and what time it is. In schizophrenia, hallucinations usually are auditory. The patients hear voices. In contrast, the hallucinations of all toxic psychoses, including those precipitated by amphetamines, are visual. The toxic psychosis associated with amphetamine usually occurs after a single very high dose.

What is of greater interest to us here is the amphetamine psychosis which takes place in addicts who have consumed large amounts of the drug gradually over a period of several days. As already mentioned, the psychosis closely mimics paranoid schizophrenia. These paranoid ideas are the hallmark of the "classic amphetamine psychosis." The delusions begin with a vague suspiciousness. As the suspiciousness increases, amphetamine users tend to develop ideas of reference— which simply means that they assume that anything which takes place in their environment has special relevance to themselves. If a fire engine passes down the street, this must have some special meaning *for them.* Since amphetamine abusers are, with good reason, fearful of the police and personal enemies, they attribute the faintest noise to people coming to get them.

The stereotyped compulsive behavior described above in amphetamine addicts tends to occur especially when they become psychotic. Patients analyze details in a concrete and repetitive manner. They have the compulsion to take objects apart, to sort, and on rare occasions put them back together. Patients pace back and forth and often move their mouth from side to side in a grimacing fashion.

William Burroughs, Jr., son of the eminent author of *Naked Lunch* and other books, spent several months of his adolescence addicted to amphetamine in the streets of Greenwich Village, New York. He wrote a book, *Speed,* recounting his experiences. While on the drug he manifested the classic stereotyped behavior,

> I went walking up and down alleys and, stoneyfaced, traced a figure eight as I walked around the two blocks . . . I flicked in and out of neon lights as I passed and repassed people . . . and I started wondering if there wasn't a jumping-off place so I could relax for a while to listen down into my own self . . . I spent the next four hours chuckling uneasily as I rerepeated the walk from West side to East wondering where to go and as to how.

The majority of patients with amphetamine psychosis experience hallucinations. Authorities differ in their estimates of the relative frequency of visual versus auditory hallucinations. Probably the discrepancies stem from confusion as whether given individuals have experienced a "classic amphetamine psychosis" resembling paranoid schizophrenia or are suffering merely from a toxic amphetamine psychosis in which visual hallucinations would be expected to occur more frequently than auditory ones. Some amphetamine users have experienced both types of psychosis. William Burroughs, Jr., reported both kinds. On one occasion, when he had taken a large amount of the drug acutely, he reported,

> I started seeing faces everywhere. No matter where I looked someone was there. Tiny people slept in my ashtray and the giant slouched, sulking, against the Chrysler Building. The trees in Washington Square were filled with faces from the past that blew in the breeze, even though I am still very young. In the mirror, my own face crawled with a dozen others making positive identification impossible, but none of this was anything to worry about, I thought, because it was just a drug reaction.

By contrast, Dr. P. H. Connell, who wrote a classic monograph compiling the detailed histories of forty-two amphetamine psychotics (a remarkable feat, since he published the study in 1956, a time when there were exceedingly few amphetamine addicts in Britain), described numerous patients with auditory hallucinations after gradually developing psychosis following repeated drug taking over a prolonged time. One man had been "taking the whole contents of an amphetamine inhaler daily for months. He began to feel that strangers were following him and heard voices talking from shop windows." Another patient "had been chewing the contents of amphetamine inhalers for twelve months. The dose had been one tube a day. He began hearing voices three weeks before admission and argued with these voices." A student "had been ingesting the contents of amphetamine inhalers for about 3 months. The evening of his admission he was convinced that everyone was trying to gas him and heard people talking about him." Thus while visual hallucinations may predominate in "toxic" amphetamine psychosis, which occurs after only a few large doses, auditory hallucinations are especially frequent among those whose psychosis has appeared more gradually. And it is the latter group whose disturbance most closely resembles paranoid schizophrenia.

Hallucinations of touch occur in amphetamine addicts, especially when they are psychotic, and seem to be closely associated with delusions of parasites beneath the skin. Patients will begin by having a sensation of tingling or itching, which then leads to examining, scratching, and rubbing the skin. As they begin to form delusions about what is taking place, they conclude that small animals, worms, lice, or crystals of amphetamine had been placed beneath their skin. This is all strikingly reminiscent of similar hallucinations of touch which we described before in cocaine addicts. It may represent another aspect of the stereotyped compulsive behavior.

Dr. Everett Ellinwood studied both human amphetamine psychotics and monkeys to whom he had chronically administered large doses of amphetamine. The monkeys would continually examine and scratch their skin much like the amphetamine addicts. Ellinwood thought that it seemed to resemble an exaggeration and a compulsive repetition of "grooming" behavior.

A key aspect of amphetamine psychosis which tends most to make me feel that it is a model schizophrenia is that it occurs in a setting of clear consciousness and correct orientation as to where the patient is located. Indeed most patients have a hyperacute memory for all events that transpired during their drug intoxication.

A Remarkable Experiment:
Driving People Mad with Amphetamine

However, before accepting the close resemblance of amphetamine psychosis to paranoid schizophrenia, we should attempt to resolve a number of serious questions. For instance, perhaps amphetamines themselves are not responsible for the psychosis; rather, some primary action of amphetamines may give rise secondarily to psychosis. Thus, with large doses of amphetamine, patients often don't sleep for several consecutive days. Perhaps amphetamine psychosis is merely a by-product of sleep deprivation. Alternatively, since amphetamines are powerful central stimulants, perhaps the psychosis is simply attributable to "overstimulation." Also, it is possible that the stimulant stress of amphetamines simply precipitates a latent form of schizophrenia. This would not be too surprising, since amphetamine addicts, the people in whom amphetamine psychosis occurs, are obviously disturbed individuals; otherwise they wouldn't be addicting themselves to amphetamines.

One way to resolve some of these questions would be to induce amphetamine psychosis experimentally in human subjects and to observe the sequence of events. Of course, deliberately inducing psychosis in humans is a rather scary business, something that would be essayed only by the most bold experimenters. During the past few years a few psychiatric researchers, after very careful and thoughtful preparation and evaluation of all the ethical considerations, conducted such studies. The major research has been undertaken by Dr. John Griffith at Vanderbilt University and Drs. Burton Angrist and Samuel Gershon at New York University. Because such experiments are so important in helping us to understand the mechanisms of amphetamine psychosis we will review in detail the results of Dr. Griffith.

Since it was not possible to obtain individuals who had never taken any drugs, Dr. Griffith recruited heavy amphetamine users. He took great care to exclude any

subjects with a prior history of amphetamine psychosis
or even the faintest indication of schizophrenic or
schizoid tendencies. The only psychiatric diagnosis of
his subjects was "moderate personality disorder,"
which is a diagnosis which any drug abusers would fit
almost by definition.

He gave his subjects dextroamphetamine sulfate in
10-milligram amounts by mouth every hour on the hour
of both day and night, as tolerated, and carefully monitored the subjects constantly. Every single one of seven
subjects sustained a definite psychosis between two
and five days after the start of the experiment. The
amount of amphetamine required to cause the psychosis ranged from 120 to 700 milligrams.

His patients responded to the first few doses of
amphetamine with a slight euphoria, but this disappeared after five to six hours, or about 50 milligrams, of
the drug. At this point his subjects all appeared somewhat depressed and began to spend much of their time
in bed, talking less, and showing little interest in watching television or reading. This is in contrast to the usual
hyperactivity of amphetamine addicts under the influence of the drug. Presumably the discrepancy is a
product of different settings. When amphetamine addicts are together they may "turn each other on," while,
in the hospital setting, subjects may well have been
depressed at the doses employed.

All the subjects lost their appetite and failed to sleep
for the first twenty-four hours. After that, those who
continued to receive amphetamines averaged about
three hours of sleep per day. Throughout the first day,
all of them were lucid and in good contact with their
environment.

About eight hours before developing explicit psychotic symptoms, the subjects became taciturn and would refuse to discuss their thoughts or feelings. Later they recall that about this time paranoid ideas began to enter their heads, but these could be dismissed with some effort as unreal and caused by the drug.

The experimenters were able to pinpoint the abrupt onset of "psychosis proper." Whereas before the subjects had been stoneyfaced and silent, now they began to discuss their thoughts openly and with animation, although in a strange, cold, and aloof manner. All of them developed well-organized paranoid ideas. One felt he was being subjected to rays from a "giant oscillator." Another maintained that he was going to be killed by his wife. After stopping the drug, the psychosis dissipated within eight hours in most of the subjects, although a few remained somewhat paranoid for another few days.

I have described this study in some detail, because it provides fairly clear answers to certain important questions. For instance, Dr. Griffith's study demonstrates that the psychosis is not simply due to sleep deprivation. Two of the subjects became psychotic on the second day, at which time amphetamine administration was stopped, so that they lost only one night of sleep. This is certainly too short a period of sleep deprivation to cause psychosis.

Careful patient selection enabled Griffith to conclude that the psychosis was not merely a drug-activated latent schizophrenia. While his subjects did have personality disorders with mild or moderate psychopathic tendencies, none had ever been schizophrenic or even showed schizoid behavior. It is also unlikely that the psychosis was a result of drug-induced arousal, because none of the subjects were at any time particularly overstimulated. In fact after the first few hours they all appeared depressed, though I must admit that observable activity may fail to reflect "internal" hyperarousal.

How Closely Does Amphetamine Psychosis Resemble Schizophrenia?

Amphetamine psychosis is not simply the precipitation of latent schizophrenia; nor is it related to sleep deprivation or central stimulation. But how much schizophrenia is it? One simple way of answering this question is simply to enumerate the large number of patients admitted to hospitals with amphetamine psychosis but misdiagnosed as paranoid schizophrenics until the history of drug use was obtained. The psychiatric literature contains well over a hundred patients misdiagnosed in this way, and we can assume that there are many others whose case histories were never published.

Another way of getting at this point is to evaluate the exact symptoms of amphetamine psychosis as contrasted to those of schizophrenia. The presence of auditory hallucinations and the fact that psychosis occurs in a setting of clear consciousness certainly favors the resemblance to schizophrenia. However, several authors have remarked that, as with cocaine psychosis, it was difficult to demonstrate the presence of the typical schizophrenic thought disturbances or feeling responses to the environment.

In the experimental studies which have been carried out, Dr. John Griffith did not feel that the classic schizophrenic thought disorder or feeling disturbance was present in his patients. Drs. Angrist and Gershon, on the other hand, reported these abnormalities in many of their patients. My own feeling is that there must be something very schizophrenic about the thinking and feeling states of these patients, since the thinking and feeling abnormalities are classically said to be the *sine qua non* for a diagnosis of schizophrenia, and we have already remarked that amphetamine psychotics are clinically indistinguishable from acute paranoid schizophrenics.

Probably the difficulty that some psychiatrists have in detecting schizophrenic thinking and feeling abnormalities in amphetamine psychotics is something like the following: Paranoid schizophrenics are individuals who have well-organized logical delusional systems. It is not at all surprising, therefore, that such individuals would often not appear to be thinking in the vague, tangential fashion traditionally associated with schizophrenia. As for the typically schizophrenic feeling abnormalities, it is well known to psychiatrists that very acute schizophrenics in the throes of their nervous breakdown often display vigorous feeling responses to the interviewer. Perhaps the confusion about the presence of these disorders in amphetamine psychotics has to do with the tendency to search for disturbances which would be characteristic of chronic schizophrenics, not of acute paranoid schizophrenics.

Other features of amphetamine psychosis also remind us of schizophrenia. Of the many drugs which have been tried out as antidotes for amphetamine psychosis, the phenothiazine tranquilizers have turned out to be uniquely effective. And, of course, these are also unique in their selective antischizophrenic action. Interestingly, since amphetamines are "uppers," addicts naturally tended to try "downers" such as barbiturates to turn off the amphetamine psychosis. However, barbiturates are not useful and even sometimes make the psychosis worse. By contrast, the phenothiazines "turn off" the amphetamine psychosis swiftly, almost as when one turns off an electric light. The more potent antischizophrenic agents tend to be most effective in relieving the symptoms of amphetamine psychosis. In animals, too, behavior disturbances elicited by amphetamine are alleviated by phenothiazine tranquilizers *in proportion to* the antischizophrenic efficacy of the drugs. Indeed, several major pharmaceutical concerns use this property, the anti-amphetamine action, as their major screening device is developing new antischizophrenic agents.

Amphetamine Makes Schizophrenia Worse

Another item, while not bearing upon amphetamine psychosis directly, does tend to associate it with schizophrenia. For many years it has been the general impression of psychiatrists in Europe and England that amphetamine in small doses can be a useful diagnostic aid for patients in whom the physician questions whether or not they are suffering from schizophrenia. A small amount of amphetamine, about 10 to 20 milligrams, will "activate" latent schizophrenic symptoms into a florid form.

Recently Dr. John Davis and his collaborators at Vanderbuilt University have demonstrated this point in straightforward experiments. They administered Ritalin, an amphetamine analogue, intravenously to patients with a variety of diagnoses. Individuals who were actively or incipiently schizophrenic developed florid symptoms. By contrast, schizophrenics in complete remission, who seemed to be fully devoid of symptoms, did not worsen with Ritalin. Depression and manic patients also failed to develop anything resembling schizophrenic symptoms with the drug.

What was most remarkable in Dr. Davis' studies was the extraordinary rapidity with which schizophrenic symptoms could be exacerbated. Witness some of his patients:

R.H., a twenty-eight-year-old schizophrenic, was admitted to the hospital complaining that "spirits" were talking to him and that he "could see and sense spirits arising out of peoples' bodies." He showed marked loosening of associations [schizophrenic thought disorder] and flattened affect [a schizophrenic disturbance of feeling processes]. Following two weeks of treatment with chlorpromazine, the patient showed a lessening of his loose associations and said that his talk about spirits was "crazy talk." Within one minute of Ritalin infusion, the patient exclaimed that the spirits had again began to talk to him and that he could see them rising out of the interviewer's head. He also showed marked loosening of associations and increased flattening of affect.

After receiving Ritalin another patient developed symptoms which were worse than she had experienced before. This twenty-six-year-old woman was withdrawn, depressed, and had a typically schizophrenic disturbance of feeling. Within one minute of Ritalin infusion, she became terrified, started screaming, and stated that she heard and saw her dead father. She then progressed into a state of extreme withdrawal with muteness and inactivity. She reported this phase of her interview retrospectively, and stated that she had paranoid thoughts and occasional hallucinations before the infusion which she had been reluctant to discuss. These had markedly increased after the drug administration. By six hours after the infusion, the patient had returned to her baseline state.

Let us then summarize the ways in which amphetamine psychosis and related states remind us of schizophrenia.

(1) Amphetamine psychosis is the only drug psychosis known (with the exception of cocaine psychosis, which is for all good purposes equivalent to amphetamine psychosis) which so closely resembles schizophrenia, of the acute paranoid type, that patients are regularly misdiagnosed as schizophrenics. This cannot be said for any other drug-induced psychosis, including the disturbances following psychedelic drugs, which are almost never mistaken for schizophrenia.

(2) The schizophrenialike symptoms of amphetamine psychosis are true drug effects and not a result of sleep loss or activation of latent schizophrenia.

(3) Phenothiazine tranquilizers are uniquely effective in treating both amphetamine psychosis and schizophrenia.

(4) Amphetamines in small doses activate the symptoms of incipient or mildly symptomatic schizophrenics but fail to have this affect on schizophrenics in remission or in manic depressed patients or normal individuals.

A Problem and Perhaps a Solution

Before leaping to any conclusions about amphetamine psychosis providing a model for understanding schizophrenia, there remains one major conundrum. Why is it that the psychosis following amphetamine use is always an acute paranoid one? Why isn't it catatonic or hebephrenic? I don't know the answer for certain. However, I have several hunches. Amphetamine is a drug. All drugs have multiple actions. Amphetamine was not cast down from heaven as a perfect "schizophrenia-producing" machine. Among the multiplicity of amphetamine actions are its ability to provoke stereotyped compulsive behavior, central stimulation, and so on. Perhaps among its many actions amphetamine does have a pure schizophrenia-mimicking property. However, other, contaminating actions of the drug confer the paranoid flavor upon the schizophrenialike psychosis.

An ideal candidate for such a "contaminating" action would be the central stimulant action of amphetamine. For what is a more commonsensical way of describing a paranoid schizophrenic then to view him as a schizophrenic who is functioning in a state of great alertness? It is the alert, centrally stimulated features of the paranoid schizophrenic's mental apparatus which probably provoke him to strive for an intellectual framework in which to focus all the strange feelings that are coming over him as the psychosis develops. This quest for meaning and its subsequent "discovery" in a system of delusions might be the essence of the paranoid process in these patients.

Conceivably, if we were able to divide the biochemical alterations in the brain which account for each of amphetamine's behavioral effects, we could tease apart the substrata for the different components of amphetamine psychosis. Perhaps one specific biochemical action wrought in people's brains by amphetamine causes central stimulation, while a completely different biochemical effect is responsible for the schizophrenialike symptoms. If so, one might, in theory, design a drug which would act selectively on the "schizophrenia" locus in the brain. With such an amphetamine derivative, one would anticipate that it would be possible to produce a model schizophrenia which would resemble an undifferentiated form of schizophrenia, or perhaps one determined by the past personality of the patient. Such a prospect gives us the motivation to go forward now and experiment with some fundamental aspects of brain function and interactions of chemicals in the brain with drugs.

11

The Brain and Its Juices

We have talked about schizophrenia at length from the psychological point of view. There is no way of knowing for certain whether schizophrenia is a single disease and, if so, whether it is produced by a unitary psychological abnormality. Many people have postulated unique, primary defects in this disease. One possible guess was that schizophrenics suffer from a defect in integrating things they perceive in their environment with their internal feelings, a complicated sort of "perceptual dysfunction."

We also spoke of drugs. Most people would agree that the phenothiazine tranquilizers and related agents do exert a selective antischizophrenic action. If we knew exactly what that action was in the brain, we might have a clue toward the fundamental disturbance in the brains of schizophrenic patients. Similarly, amphetamine and cocaine can elicit psychoses which are clinically indistinguishable from some forms of schizophrenia. Moreover, in low doses amphetamine can "activate" a quiescent schizophrenic in a fairly specific fashion. This suggests that the biochemical key to these effects of amphetamine should shed light upon the chemical basis of schizophrenia.

Now we are ready for the impossible, or what is almost impossible—to tie all of these lines of evidence together. For this endeavor we must review what the different parts of the brain generally have to do with various emotional states. Then, we will attempt to explain a few key biochemical features of brain function, especially the critical process called "neurotransmission." Next, we will talk about what we know of just how drugs such as the phenothiazines and amphetamines exert their characteristic effects upon man's emotional state. And finally we will judge what, if anything, this tells us about schizophrenia.

Man Has Many Brains

The human brain, or for that matter the brain of almost any animal, is a strange-looking device, even when viewed without a microscope and even when one looks only at its external surface, as depicted in Figure 1. There really seem to be several brains. The most striking part of the human brain is the cerebral cortex which surmounts the whole affair and is replete with many convolutions and fissures. Just as the cerebral cortex is the "top" of the brain, so the brain stem is at the bottom. The brain stem appears almost to be no more than a fattened upward extension of the spinal cord. As the brain stem ascends it merges into the

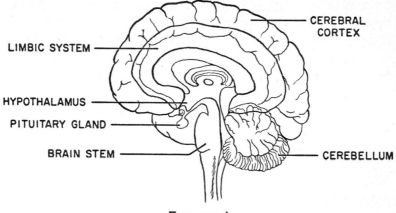

FIGURE 1

hypothalamus, a relatively small but crucial structure which connects the brain stem to the cerebral cortex more or less, and which is itself connected not only to the rest of the brain but also to the pituitary gland, the "master" gland of the entire body. Encircling the brain stem and hypothalamus just beneath the major part of the cerebral cortex is the "limbic system," which can be considered part of the cerebral cortex but which, in fact, differs from most of it in terms of function and origin.

One way of viewing the functions of the brain is to recognize that they become more "sophisticated" or "modern" as one ascends from the spinal cord. Indeed, this is the way the brain evolved through history from the lowest animals to man. The spinal cord is the most primitive area. It can "mastermind" a few simple muscle reflexes, but for the most part only transmits information from higher centers down to the rest of the body or conveys sensations upward.

The brain stem is a critical regulatory center for many primitive but essential body functions. Here are contained centers controlling breathing and the heart-beat. Therefore, damage to the brain stem by tumor, blood clot, or trauma is more rapidly and certainly fatal than damage to any other part of the brain. In fact, tumors or blood clots in other areas of the brain often kill the victim simply because they squeeze the affected portion of the brain and the mechanical pressures are transmitted to the brain stem. Besides these fundamental processes, the brain stem has other very important functions. Within the brain stem is contained the "reticular activating system." This is an intricate meshwork of nerves which plays a crucial role in regulating awareness. Damage to the reticular activating system can plunge an animal or man immediately into profound and irreversible coma. An electrical stimulation of the reticular activating system in a somnolent animal quickly rouses him to an alert state.

The cerebellum looks like a completely separate part of the brain; like a little brain unto itself. When the cerebellum is examined under the microscope it appears to be organized in a more systematic or machine-like fashion than any other portion of the brain. Indeed, most neurophysiologists feel that its role is to act very much like a complex computer with all sorts of feedback loops to modulate the commands of the cerebral cortex and other portions of the brain having to do with movement of the arms and legs. The cerebellum insures that these movements will be smooth and well coordinated.

The hypothalamus has important functions in controlling the state of the internal body organs. For instance, electrical stimulation in the hypothalamus can alter the heart rate. Moreover, the pituitary gland is directly controlled by the hypothalamus, which secretes hormones into a collection of small blood vessels that connect the hypothalamus and the pituitary gland. These very special hormones, called "releasing factors," migrate in the blood vessels to the pituitary gland, where they activate the release of the important hormones of the pituitary gland. These latter hormones then go into the general circulation and "turn on" glands throughout the body, including the adrenal gland, the thyroid gland, and the male and female gonads.

The hypothalamus also has much to do with emotions. Almost twenty years ago James Olds at the University of Michigan showed that part of the hypothalamus can function as a "pleasure center." In Olds's classic experiment, electrodes were implanted in the lateral part of the hypothalamus of rats and connected by a series of wires to a lever, such that when the rat pressed the lever he delivered an electrical shock to his hypothalamus. If the electrode is in the appropriate location, such rats will press the lever at a furious rate, thousands of times in an hour, in order to deliver shocks to their hypothalami. Presumably such shocks must "feel good." In the hypothalamus there are also specialized "hunger" and "satiety" centers. If a rat's hunger center is destroyed, he loses all interest in food and may literally starve to death. By contrast, destruction of the satiety center produces a glutton of a rat, who eats ravenously and becomes extraordinarily obese.

The limbic system contains a number of structures with somewhat differing functions, but all of which have in common features related to emotions and memory. The destruction of certain parts of the limbic system can produce a peculiar sort of memory impairment. The individual can remember what he has to do on a very short-term basis. Thus if one reads off to him rapidly a sequence of items to purchase in the store, he can do this if he goes down the list rapidly. However, if distracted even for a brief interval, he can no longer recall it.

Emotional functions of the limbic system are of greatest interest to us here. Electrical stimulation of part of the limbic system can produce ferocious rage in animals. Destruction of such areas results in a very docile animal. Alterations in certain portions of the limbic system have a variety of effects on sexual behavior. Appropriate manipulations can produce hypersexuality, lack of sexual interest, or even "perverted" sexual behavior.

The cerebral cortex seems to be the boss of everything else. Within the cerebral cortex are located "language" centers which control all aspects of speech and the handling of language. People who have suffered strokes in these areas of the brain manifest one of a number of forms of "aphasia," a word derived from *phasis,* the Greek term for speech, and which refers to a loss of the power of expression or comprehension of written or spoken language. Within the cerebral cortex are centers for the subtle discrimination of sensation. Loss of the "visual" portion of the cerebral cortex results in an interesting form of blindness. Though the patient cannot see, he may respond to environmental stimulation, because the visual sensation reaches lower centers of the brain.

Information for the various modes of perception reaches the cerebral cortex via thick lengthy brain tracts, some of which contain nerves that course unimpeded all the way from the sensory organ to the cerebral cortex. Through these large and well-insulated tracks, sensory information travels at extraordinary speed to the cerebral cortex. It was originally thought that this was all there was to sensation. However, about twenty years ago it became evident that collateral nerves from the sensory pathways enter the brain stem, diverging from the main path which proceeds essentially nonstop to the cerebral cortex, and in the brain stem becomes intermingled with a vast network of small nerves within the reticular activating system. Via these collaterals, events perceived in the environment may be integrated with information already stored within the brain, and with internal bodily sensations, information about which arises up through the spinal cord and into the brain stem and hypothalamus. Similarly, the perceptual information may be integrated with emotional states encoded in the hypothalamus and limbic system. These interactions presumably convey an emotional, "gut" component to every perception. Once the perception is stored as a "memory," we can assume that the memory is "tagged" with these associated feeling states. In this way man does not function like an unfeeling electronic computer. Instead, every memory and every perception has an associated feeling or "affective" component. What the organism does about stimuli which he has perceived depends as much on the gut component of the perception as on its intellectual informational component.

Nerves and Their Connections

How is information processed by these various areas of the brain? The fundamental unit in the brain, as in the rest of the body, is the cell. A cell is a walled-off unit containing the essential ingredients of life: a nucleus with DNA, the genetic material; machinery to manufacture proteins, fats, and carbohydrates; and a cell membrane which regulates contact between the inside of the cell and the outside world in a very dynamic fashion. The brain contains two kinds of cells: nerve cells or "neurons" and glial cells. Though there will always be controversy about the exact function of the glial cells, most scientists feel that they are primarily the supporting cast for the prima donna neurons. Interestingly, there are more glial cells than neurons in the brain. Very recent research suggests that, though the glial cells may be subservient to the neurons, they may play an active role in modulating the functions of the neurons.

Neurons differ from other cells in the body in that they are extremely excitable and possess long extensions called axons or dendrites, as depicted in Figure 2. The electrical state of the membrane of neurons can be altered; and when excited, a "nerve impulse," which is quite analogous to an electric current carried by a wire, passes down the length of the neuron. In contrast to an electric wire in which the current is carried by the passage of electrons, nerve impulses are carried along nerve fibers by a flow of metal ions, especially sodium. Nerve impulses generally flow in only one direction. Information regarding the nerve impulse originates in the dendrites, which are the "antennae" or receiving elements for the neuron. The cell body is comparable to the totality of most cells and contains a nucleus and all the machinery for protein manufacture. The axon is the long fiber which can travel any distance from a fraction of a millimeter to a foot, depending on the nature of the particular neuron. The nerve ending is literally that area where the axon terminates.

Of great importance is the fact that in the brain most axons split up near their termination into a vast multitude of nerve endings, each of which can influence a

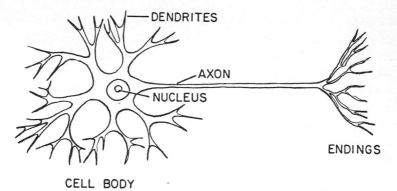

FIGURE 2

different neuron. Dendrites are similarly branched, so that a given neuron can receive information from a large number of other neurons. If a given neuron received information via its dendrites from 100 other neurons and transmitted information through its nerve endings to another 100 neurons, then that single nerve would be in a position to set up 100 times 100, or 10,000, discrete lines of communication. It is this capacity of neurons to enter into multiple and complex interactions that accounts for the almost unlimited scope that the brain processes for information transmission.

Neurotransmitters:
The Juice of Information Transmission

How do the various nerves "talk" to each other? How are messages transmitted across the gap between the nerve ending of one neuron and the dendrites or cell body of another? This space is called the "synapse." When neurophysiologists first appreciated that nerve impulses were conducted electrically, they simply assumed that the nerve impulse, like a spark, jumped across the synaptic cleft. It is now known that only in a very few synapses in the nervous system can such electrical transmission take place. For the majority, it is a physical impossibility. Instead, when the nerve impulses reach the nerve endings, they trigger the release of a specialized chemical, called a neurotransmitter, which then diffuses across the synaptic cleft and transmits information to the succeeding neuron. The information transmitted can be one of two types: either the neurotransmitter is "excitatory," in which case the message is "fire," while if the neurotransmitter is "inhibitory" the message is "do not fire."

Several different neutrotransmitters operate in the brain, how many we do not know. However, it seems that a given neuron uses only a single neurotransmitter. Some neurotransmitters may be capable only of conveying either excitatory or inhibitory information, but never both; while others may be excitatory at certain synapses and inhibitory at others. Scientists still have no idea as to just what makes a neurotransmitter inhibitory or excitatory. Indeed, they haven't the faintest notion as to the nature of the interaction between the neurotransmitter and the membrane of the neuron upon which it acts that can account for the change in the electrical properties of this membrane. It is still a very mysterious business.

Catecholamines:
Neurotransmitters of Emotion?

Thought there may be ten or more different classes of neurotransmitters, in order to explain what seems to be the most interesting and potentially significant interactions of drugs, neurotransmitters, and schizophrenia, we will focus only on a couple of neurotransmitters and describe the other known ones in an appendix.

The neutrotransmitters of particular interest are collectively called the "catecholamines." Catecholamine is a term which describes the chemical make-up of norepinephrine and dopamine, the neurotransmitters of specific interest. Norepinephrine and dopamine are closely related chemically; both are called catecholamines because of their chemical structure. They are sufficiently similar that in many parts of the brain where norepinephrine is the predominent catecholamine neurotransmitter, dopamine serves as its precursor. By this I mean that norepinephrine is formed by a chemical transformation of dopamine. In certain parts of the brain, however, there is little or no norepinephrine but considerable amounts of dopamine; and in these brain regions dopamine is the catecholamine neurotransmitter.

In general, when an anatomist looks at the brain under a light microscope or electron microscope he sees many neurons. However, he has no way of knowing which neurotransmitter is localized in which neuron. To obtain such information he would need some specialized stain which would stain only one neurotransmitter and not any others. Such stains are not available for most neurotransmitters. However, we are fortunate with the catecholamines, since about ten years ago a group of Swedish scientists developed such a staining technique for the norepinephrine and dopamine.

Specifically, when brain specimens are treated with a specially prepared formaldehyde vapor, norepinephrine and dopamine develop an intense green fluorescence which can be readily visualized under the microscope. Unfortunately, this technique cannot yet be applied to the electron microscope, which can detect much smaller structures than can the light microscope. By a variety of technical maneuvers, one can distinguish between norepinephrine and dopamine. Because of this intense green fluorescence, the anatomist can now look at the brain and identify which neurons contain dopamine, which contain norepinephrine, and which contain neither. He can follow the course of these neurons throughout the brain. He can locate their cell bodies and trace out the pathway of their axons up to the nerve endings. What these techniques have revealed is that norepinephrine and dopamine neurons cluster in well-defined groups. Such clusters of neurons coursing throughout the brain together are called "brain tracts." Just by knowing the detailed geography of the various norepinephrine and dopamine tracts, one can make certain reasonable inferences as to the function of these tracts. Certain of these inferences have already borne important fruit in the treatment of certain diseases.

Dopamine and Parkinson's Disease

The most prominent dopamine tract in the brain has its cell bodies in a very discrete location within the brain stem called the substantia nigra. Its axon ascends through the brain stem and gives rise to nerve endings predominantly in the corpus striatum. The corpus striatum is a portion of the brain which we did not mention before in our classification, since it doesn't fit well into any of the defined classes. To a certain extent it seems to be part of the limbic system of structures. It has been evident to scientists who have stimulated it electrically or destroyed portions of it that the corpus striatum has

ASCENDING NOREPINEPHRINE PATHWAYS

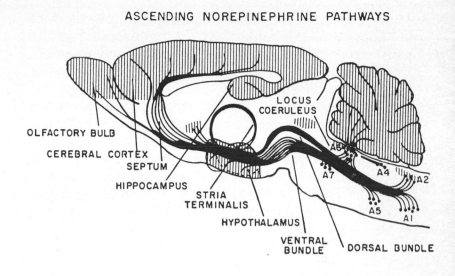

DOPAMINE PATHWAYS

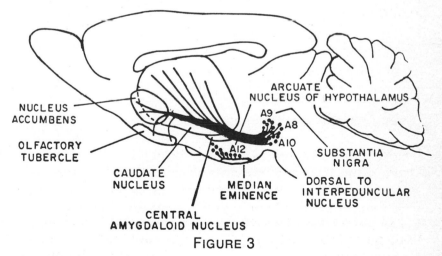

FIGURE 3

something to do with the integration of movements of the body. Until the dopamine tract that passes from the substantia nigra to the corpus striatum was discovered, many people did not appreciate that these two parts of the brain had anything to do with each other.

Dopamine and the corpus striatum have attracted national attention because of their role in Parkinson's disease. Parkinson's disease is a condition which afflicts and severely debilitates up to a million Americans every year. For some unknown reason, these patients gradually develop a stiffness of their arms and legs and face so that it is difficult to move or evince lively facial expressions. Ultimately such patients are confined to wheelchairs. Besides their inability to move, patients with Parkinson's disease suffer from a tremor of the limbs, which is especially evident in the hands.

Pathologists who examined the brains of patients dying with Parkinson's disease had been impressed that there was degeneration primarily in two parts of the brain, the corpus striatum and the substantia nigra. When the dopamine pathway connecting the substantia nigra and the corpus striatum was discovered, a number of scientists wondered whether some abnormality in dopamine in these two parts of the brain might be related to the symptoms of the disease.

The Viennese physician Dr. Oleh Hornykiewicz attacked the problem in a rather direct fashion. He obtained the brains of patients who had died of Parkinson's disease as soon as possible after their death, as well as brains of patients of a similar age but who had died of some other condition. Hornykiewicz simply measured the dopamine content of the brain in both groups. He was astounded to find that the brains of patients with Parkinson's disease were severely depleted of dopamine. They had almost none at all, especially if their Parkinson's disease had been symptomatically severe. This strongly suggested to him that the dopamine deficiency might well have something to do with the symptoms of Parkinson's disease.

However, if we think about these various items of information for a moment, we should recognize that one must be cautious before leaping to such a conclusion. Although the dopamine pathway connecting the substantia nigra and the corpus striatum is the largest of all the catecholamine pathways in the brain, it is not the most prominent collection of neurons in the corpus striatum. Indeed, of all the nerve terminals within the corpus striatum, only fifteen percent are dopamine nerve endings. Since we know that there is major degeneration of the corpus striatum in Parkinson's disease, the dopamine deficiency that Hornykiewicz discovered might only be a secondary manifestation of degeneration of the entire corpus striatum. Perhaps all the neurotransmitters in the corpus striatum would be depleted. Unfortunately, since we are ignorant of the identity of all the neurotransmitters in the brain, we cannot answer this question definitively.

Several scientists attempted an approach to determine whether the dopamine deficiency in Parkinson's disease has anything to do in a casual way with the symptoms. They reasoned simply enough that, if one were to eliminate the dopamine deficiency—that is, to restore the missing dopamine—and if such a maneuver were to relieve the symptoms, one could conclude that lack of dopamine had been responsible for the symptoms of Parkinson's disease. Unfortunately, one cannot administer dopamine directly to patients, at least not by mouth or injection outside of the brain, because dopamine has difficulty entering the brain. For one thing, it is rapidly destroyed in the liver. For another, because it is electrically charged there is a sort of "barrier" to its entering the brain. However, one can circumvent this barrier simply by giving the metabolic precusor of dopamine, L-dopa, whose proper name is L-dihydroxyphenylalanine.

L-dopa is the naturally occurring chemical in the body which is normally converted by the brain into dopamine. In contrast to dopamine, L-dopa can enter the brain when administered to the patient by mouth or injection. Since it is destroyed in the liver to a marked extent, one must give fairly large doses. Initial experiments with small doses of L-dopa were unsuccessful. However, about 1967 Dr. George Cotzias administered massive doses of L-dopa by mouth to patients with Parkinson's disease. Their symptoms were dramatically alleviated. L-dopa was far more successful than any other medication had ever been in Parkinson's disease. Indeed, it counts as one of the miracle drugs of the century. Patients who had been confined for years to wheelchairs could now move about freely. And, of theoretical importance, one could conclude that the therapeutic effectiveness of L-dopa in Parkinson's disease "proved" that the deficiency of dopamine was responsible for the symptoms of the disease.

In addition, Swedish scientist Urban Ungerstedt has obtained evidence that the dopamine pathway connecting the substantia nigra and corpus striatum is also intimately associated with and, in fact, may be a major component of the various eating centers in the hypothalamus. The dopamine fibers connecting the substantia nigra and corpus striatum pass through that portion of the hypothalamus whose destruction normally causes rats to stop eating.

When most scientists examine the functions of different portions of the brain they literally "burn" holes in the part of the brain they wish to destroy. With this technique one destroys all the neurons in a given area of the brain. The neurons destroyed may be a diverse lot, using rather different neurotransmitters. One doesn't know if the effects observed were related to all neurons or only to a particular class of the neurons within that portion of the brain. Urban Ungerstedt was able to make use of a unique drug, 6-hydroxydopamine, which selectively destroys only dopamine or norepinephrine neurons. 6-hydroxydopamine is a labile chemical which oxidizes readily and can destroy almost any sort of cell. However, since it is chemically related to dopamine and norepinephrine, it is accumulated almost exclusively by dopamine and norepinephrine neurons so that, when used in appropriate doses, these are the only types of neurons which it destroys. When Ungerstedt injects a tiny amount of 6-hydroxydopamine directly into the substantia nigra, the only part of the brain destroyed is the dopamine cells within the substantia nigra. Then the axon and nerve endings degenerate over a period of a few days. In this way, Dr. Ungerstedt is able to obliterate the dopamine pathway connecting the substantia nigra and corpus striatum without affecting any other part of the brain or any other type of neurons.

Ungerstedt selectively destroyed this particular dopamine pathway on both sides of the brain and noticed that his rats would not eat or drink. This is just what happens when one "burns out" the well-known eating centers in the hypothalamus. Ungerstedt showed that the dopamine axons passing through the hypothalamus on their way to the corpus striatum accounted for the refusal to eat that followed upon destruction of this part of the hypothalamus. Thus, besides having something to do with coordination of movements of the extremities, this fascinating dopamine pathway has something to do with regulating eating and drinking.

OTHER CATECHOLAMINE TRACTS

There are several other dopamine tracts in the brain whose function is less well understood then the one we just discussed. One dopamine tract connects the hypothalamus with the plexus of blood vessels which supplies the pituitary gland and which, as we described earlier, carries the "releasing factors" from the hypothalamus to the pituitary gland. Several scientists have experimented with this particular dopamine pathway and feel that it may play a major role in controlling the relationship of the releasing factors of the hypothalamus and their effects on the pituitary gland.

There are also dopamine pathways whose cell bodies are also in the brain stem fairly near the substantia nigra, and whose axons ascend to give off nerve endings in certain portions of the limbic system of the brain, especially the olfactory tubercle and the nucleus accumbens. These two parts of the brain are very little understood, although it has been thought for years that they have something to do with emotional behavior. Indeed in lower animals almost all of the limbic system of the brain was related to olfactory function. "Olfactory" means "related to smelling."

In animals lower than man, smelling is an extremely important sense, as we well know from our pet dogs, the best example being bloodhounds who can track down humans from a distance of miles, knowing no more than a little about their body odor as gleaned from a few sniffs at their clothing. In higher species, as the olfactory sense has become less important for survival that portion of the brain has tended to play a more prominent role in emotional behavior. As is obvious from its name, the olfactory tubercle in lower mammals plays a definite function in integrating information obtained by the smelling sense. The nucleus accumbens is located in the spinal part of the limbic system of the brain. Interestingly, it is in this spectal region that the Louisiana psychiatrists, Dr. Robert Heath some twenty years ago obtained dramatic electrical recordings of schizophrenic patients. He was audacious enough to implant electrodes into different parts of the brains of very severely chronic schizophrenic patients. From electrodes in the septal area, which includes the nucleus accumbens, he obtained abnormal spiking electrical activity which he did not observe in the septal area of other, nonschizophrenic patients.

There exist at least two major norepinephrine pathways in the brain. One is called the dorsal pathway because it tends to lie more in the dorsal part of the brain, which is that part of the brain closer to the back of the animal. The other norepinephrine pathway is called the ventral pathway, since it lies closer to the ventral surface, or that surface which would be nearer to the face side of the animal. All the cell bodies of the dorsal norepinephrine pathway are located in one discrete part of the brain stem called the locus coeruleus, or "blue place."

The name is an apt one, because when one slices through the brain and looks at the locus coeruleus, it appears to be colored blue. Axons arising from the norepinephrine cell bodies in the locus coeruleus take a number of different trips. Some of them turn downward and enter the cerebellum, the portion of the brain which is concerned with very rapid and fine coordination of motor movement. This function of the cerebellum contrasts with that of the corpus striatum which seems to regulate grosser movements of the arms and legs. Other norepinephrine fibers arising from the locus coeruleus ascend all the way up to the cerebral cortex where they branch out and influence almost all parts of the cerebral cortex.

The cell bodies of origin for the ventral norepinephrine pathway are scattered throughout several parts of the brain stem. Their axons come together and ascend along the more ventral surface of the brain stem and pass as a fairly thick bundle through the more lateral part of the hypothalamus. Within the hypothalamus they give off a number of nerve endings, while some fibers continue upward and give off further nerve endings in the limbic system. Interestingly, the location of the major norepinephrine fibers and nerve endings in the lateral hypothalamus coincides very closely with the locations where electrode placement will cause a maximal amount of self-stimulation in rats. In other words, the norepinephrine fibers and endings in the lateral hypothalamus seem to be localized discretely in the pleasure centers. A number of experiments in which levels of norepinephrine have been elevated or depressed by various manipulations strongly suggests that the norepinephrine fibers and endings in the lateral hypothalamus are essential components of the pleasure center. Thus we can surmise that the major function of the ventral norepinephrine pathway has to do with regulation of pleasurable feelings, with euphoria, elation, and presumably also with feelings of depression.

STOPPING NEUROTRANSMITTER ACTIONS AT SYNAPSES

Information processing at synapses must take place quite rapidly to maintain the mental functioning of the average human being—functioning which, if we think about it for a moment, must be taking place at break-neck speed. Therefore, after a neurotransmitter crosses the synaptic cleft and excites or inhibits the next neuron, one would want to get rid of the transmitter expeditiously so that the neuron can be prepared for succeeding nerve impulses. At least two specialized mechanisms for freeing the synaptic cleft of transmitter are relatively well known. The first discovered was a process whereby the transmitter is physically destroyed by an enzyme. Enzymes are protein molecules which catalyze chemical reactions in the body: which is to say that they make these reactions occur efficiently and speedily. Certain neurotransmitters are destroyed by enzymes that are highly localized to an area close by the sites where the transmitter excites or inhibits the neuron.

Synaptic actions of the catecholamines norepinephrine and dopamine are terminated in an entirely different way. After they have acted on the membrane receptor sites, norepinephrine and dopamine are almost literally pumped back into the nerve ending which had released them, as depicted in Figure 4. They are "taken up" into these nerve endings by a process which requires considerable energy and can operate rapidly and effectively even at the low concentrations of norepinephrine which are presumably present in the synaptic cleft. The eminent pharmacologist Julius Axelrod and his collaborators deserve a great deal of the credit for discovering this unique means for terminating the

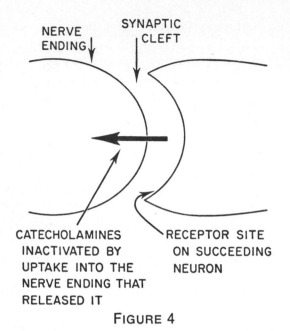

NERVE
ENDING

SYNAPTIC
CLEFT

CATECHOLAMINES
INACTIVATED BY
UPTAKE INTO THE
NERVE ENDING THAT
RELEASED IT

RECEPTOR SITE
ON SUCCEEDING
NEURON

FIGURE 4

synaptic activities of neurotransmitters; this discovery, in part, was responsible for the awarding of the Nobel Prize in medicine and physiology to Axelrod in 1970.

Otto Loewi in the late 1920s made the epochal discovery that information transmission across synapses was mediated via chemicals released by nerves. Loewi also played a role in showing that enzymes can destroy the neurotransmitter after its release into the synaptic cleft. Working with acetylcholine, the first-known neurotransmitter, he discovered evidence that an enzyme destroyed acetylcholine shortly after its release into the synaptic cleft. Thus, as early as 1930 people assumed that enzymatic destruction accounted for the termination of synaptic activities of neurotransmitters. This view was so ingrained in the thinking of brain scientists that when Julius Axelrod, about 1960, proposed that the synaptic actions of norepinephrine might be terminated by "re-uptake" of norepinephrine into the nerve endings that had released it, his proposal was greeted with great skepticism on the part of most students of the brain. However, in the past decade it has become more and more evident that this re-uptake process may be even more important than Axelrod first thought.

Not only are norepinephrine and dopamine removed from the synaptic cleft by re-uptake into the nerve endings that had released them, but this re-uptake process seems to be a universal mechanism for an activation of neurotransmitters. Almost every neuro- transmitter not known appears to be inactivated by analogous re-uptake processes. The neuron which con- tains each neurotransmitter has its own highly specific re-uptake process for its very own transmitter. Acetyl- choline appears to be virtually the only major neuro- transmitter for which there is no re-uptake system. Therefore, its inactivation via destruction by an enzyme now appears to be an exception to the general rule that neurotransmitters are inactivated via re-uptake. A varie- ty of drugs may exert their therapeutic actions via effects produced upon these re-uptake processes. Some of these may be important for our understanding of norepinephrine and dopamine and their interactions via drugs.

12

Drugs
and the Brain
and Schizophrenia

With this brief background about neurotransmitter disposition in the brain, we may be in a position to explore how some of the drugs which are important to understanding schizophrenia exert their therapeutic effects. The phenothiazine tranquilizers provided our first major clue to a relationship between brain chemistry and the symptoms of schizophrenia. How do they act?

When one examines the chemical formulae of the phenothiazine drugs, one does not detect any obvious resemblance to any known chemicals in the brain, be they neurotransmitter or not. Thus, for a number of years after introduction of the phenothiazines scientists were in a quandary as to how these important drugs might do their job. There was no dearth of research activity. Every brain scientist, be he biochemist, pharmacologist, or neurophysiologist, thought chlorpromazine had effects upon almost every system studied. This is not at all surprising, for, if one looks at the chlorpromazine molecule, it is evident that it is a highly reactive chemical that would interact in a variety of ways with all manner of brain and general body constituents. Thus the neurophysiologist found that chlorpromazine would alter the firing rate of almost every neuron examined. Biochemists who studied the respiration of brain tissue—namely, its ability to oxidize and derive energy from foodstuffs—found that chlorpromazine had powerful influences upon respiration. Chlorpromazine even has direct physical effects upon parts of cells. It can cause mitochondria, the energy-producing particles within cells, to swell.

Naturally, each scientist who discovered one or another of these effects of chlorpromazine suggested that *their* effect might be the one which was ultimately responsible for the antischizophrenic action of the phenothiazines. How is one to choose between the modes of actions of the drug? Pharmacologists confront this sort of dilemma almost daily with all sorts of drugs. For it is a truism in pharmacology that no drug is entirely specific in its actions. All drugs have diverse effects on many systems, only one of which is responsible for their therapeutic effectiveness. The dilemma is the same, only a little more complicated in total dimension, with the phenothiazines. Of course, though it may be more difficult to pinpoint the therapeutically meaningful actions of the phenothiazines, the payoff in terms of our understanding of the brain and schizophrenia is proportionately greater.

There is at least one productive approach to determining the relevance of particular biochemical actions of the phenothiazines. Among the many phenothiazines and related antischizophrenic drugs, there exist a number of striking variations in potency. For instance, haloperidol is a drug of the butyrophenone class which, though different chemically from the phenothiazines, has essentially the same sorts of therapeutic actions in schizophrenic patients. Haloperidol is about 100 times as potent as chlorpromazine in human subjects. Thus a dose of 1 milligram of haloperidol will have about the same therapeutic effect as 100 milligrams of chlopromazine. If a given action of the phenothiazines is thought to be relevant to the antischizophrenic actions of these drugs, then one would expect haloperidol to be considerably more potent than chlorpromazine in eliciting such an effect.

Similarly, as we discussed in earlier chapters, some phenothiazines, though quite similar chemically to chlorpromazine, have no antischizophrenic reactions at all. The drug promethazine, whose trade name is Phenergan, is a very widely used antihistamine and is a phenothiazine, but it is not at all effective in schizophrenia. Again, any biochemical action of phenothiazines which has a meaningful relationship to their effects in schizophrenia should be exerted by chlorpromazine but not by promethazine.

When one goes through the multiplicity of different neurophysiological and biochemical actions of chlorpromazine described in hundreds and even thousands of publications, almost all of them flunk the simple test of relevance cited above. For virtually all of the effects, promethazine is just as effective as chlorpromazine. Moreover, there is little or no correlation between the antischizophrenic potency of the phenothiazines and their ability to elicit most biochemical and neurophysiological actions. There is, however, one exception to this record of failure.

In 1963, eleven years after chlorpromazine was first employed in psychiatric patients, the Swedish pharmacologist Arvid Carlsson published a short paper describing some effects of chlorpromazine on the rate of destruction of dopamine and norepinephrine in the brain. These effects were not particularly dramatic, but they satisfied the important criteria we set out above. Chlorpromazine was effective; haloperidol was almost a hundred times as potent as chlorpromazine; and promethazine was devoid of any effect. On the basis of his fairly meager biochemical data, Carlsson speculated as to what action the phenothiazines were exerting upon dopamine and norepinephrine neurons. He suggested that these drugs block the receptor sites for dopamine and norepinephrine, as depicted in Figure 1.

These receptor sites presumably are specialized locations on the membranes of neurons where nerve endings from dopamine or norepinephrine neurons terminate. Such receptor sites are thought to be highly specialized for receiving norepinephrine or dopamine molecules in a very specific lock-and-key arrangement so that the neurotransmitter–receptor interaction can thereupon trigger a change in the electrical properties of the neuron. Carlsson proposed that norepinephrine and dopamine block these receptor sites thus preventing the access of dopamine or norepinephrine molecules.

Something within the neuron recognizes this sudden absence of neurotransmitter molecules at their appropriate receptor site and one way or another transmits a message back to the norepinephrine or dopamine neurons saying something like the following, "We don't have enough norepinephrine or dopamine. Please send us some more!" Whereupon the norepinephrine or dopamine neuron in question proceeds to fire

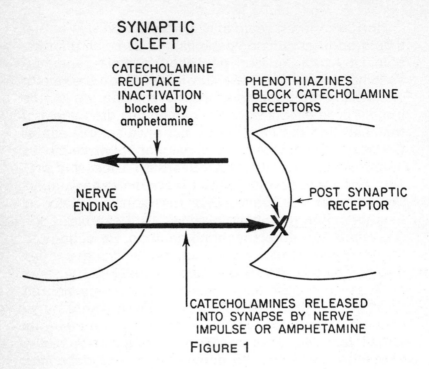

SYNAPTIC
CLEFT

CATECHOLAMINE
REUPTAKE
INACTIVATION
blocked by
amphetamine

PHENOTHIAZINES
BLOCK CATECHOLAMINE
RECEPTORS

NERVE
ENDING

POST SYNAPTIC
RECEPTOR

CATECHOLAMINES RELEASED
INTO SYNAPSE BY NERVE
IMPULSE OR AMPHETAMINE

FIGURE 1

at a more rapid rate. Naturally, when it fires more frequently it discharges more norepinephrine or dopamine molecules and accordingly must manufacture brand new norepinephrine or dopamine molecules to make up for those which are lost when they are released from the nerve endings. (Although some norepinephrine and dopamine molecules are conserved by reuptake of molecules that have been released, a goodly portion escape the re-uptake process.) Accordingly, along with the acceleration of the firing rates of norepinephrine and dopamine neurons, one obtains an enhanced formation of new norepinephrine and dopamine molecules.

With the greater release of norepinephrine and

dopamine into the synaptic cleft, one would also anticipate the formation of greater quantities of breakdown
products of norepinephrine and dopamine. Indeed,
Carlsson's initial biochemical observation was simply
an increase in the quantity of breakdown products of
dopamine and norepinephrine after rats were treated
with chlorpromazine. The rest of the conceptual
scheme I have just described, receptor blockade by the
phenothiazines and the feedback information demand-
ing accelerated firing of dopamine and norepinephrine
neurons, was all hypothesized by Carlsson. What is
especially remarkable is Arvid Carlsson's skill as a
prophet. For he seems to have been right on all counts.

In the succeeding ten years, several scientists have
documented that there is indeed an increased formation
of norepinephrine and dopamine after animals are treated with phenothiazine drugs. Moreover, Dr. George
Aghajanian at Yale University has shown that the firing
rate of dopamine neurons is markedly enhanced after
animals are treated with phenothiazines, and he has
even been able to acquire direct biochemical evidence
that the phenothiazines do in fact block dopamine
receptors. In all of these "follow up" studies which have
confirmed and extended the original work of Carlsson;
the strict standards he set up for antischizophrenic
relevance have all been met. In all cases there is a close
parallel between antischizophrenic potency of drugs
and their ability to exert these effects upon dopamine
and norepinephrine neurons. Moreover, the phenothiazine agents which are not antischizophrenic
drugs do not exert any of the effects.

As all these new findings have accumulated and as
more and more phenothiazines and butyrophenone
tranquilizers have been examined, it has become clear
that the ability of the antischizophrenic drugs to block

dopamine receptors correlated exceedingly well with their antischizophrenic effectiveness. Actions of the drugs on norepinephrine receptors is much weaker and does not correlate nearly so well with therapeutic results in schizophrenia. Moreover, in the last few years some extraordinarily potent butyrophenone tranquilizers have been manufactured, whose antischizophrenic potency is even several times greater than that of haloperidol. With these presumably highly specific antischizophrenic drugs, essentially no effects are observed upon norepinephrine neurons. These drugs appear to be selective dopamine receptor blocking agents.

Thus there is an extremely impressive correlation between the ability of phenothiazine and butyrophenone drugs to block dopamine receptor sites in the brain and their antischizophrenic potency. It is quite tempting then to speculate that the antischizophrenic action of these drugs is mediated via blockade of dopamine receptor sites in the brain. Which of the dopamine tracts might be the best candidate for being the precise locus of the action of the phenothiazines in schizophrenia? This is an enticing and important issue. As far as we can tell, phenothiazines block dopamine receptors to a similar extent at all the dopamine pathways. To determine which has the closest relationship to the antischizophrenic actions of the drugs will require much further research. However, there is one action of phenothiazines in schizophrenic and other patients which is easier to tackle.

The most prominent side effect of these drugs is their ability to produce symptoms closely resembling those of Parkinson's disease. And, as we discussed earlier, the naturally occurring Parkinson's disease seems to be caused by a degeneration of a particular dopamine tract, namely, the one connecting the substantia nigra and the corpus striatum. Since phenothiazine drugs block dopamine receptors, they might thereby elicit a situation which, for all practical purposes, is equivalent to dopamine deficiency. The relative potency of phenothiazine drugs in eliciting Parkinsonian-like side effects closely parallels their known ability to block dopamine receptors. Indeed, most researchers are fairly well convinced that the side effects resembling Parkinson's disease are produced by a blockade of the dopamine receptors located in the corpus striatum.

Even though we have made a strong case that the phenothiazines exert their antischizophrenic action by a blockade of some dopamine receptors in the brain, we should be cautious before making the next conceptual leap to the conclusion that this effect directly reverses what is biochemically abnormal in the brains of schizophrenics. In other words, we should not hastily assert that, because blocking dopamine receptors causes therapeutic improvements in schizophrenics, schizophrenics therefore suffer primarily from an excess of dopamine in certain sites in the brain. The reason that we must be cautious is that there are alternative explanations.

The dopamine receptor sites which the phenothiazines block may not be directly related to schizophrenic abnormality, but may represent only a secondary site several steps removed from the primary abnormality in schizophrenia. However, conceivably by blocking the dopamine receptors the drugs can ease the distress of the patients so that the schizophrenic symptoms, whose primary locus is elsewhere in the brain, can "heal themselves." This would be analogous to applying a tourniquet upstream from a site of bleeding, slowing the gush of blood from a wound so that the body's clotting mechanisms could then relieve the primary abnormality, a tear in the wall of a blood vessel.

There are actually some reasons to favor an indirect action of the phenothiazines in schizophrenia. Remember that these drugs do not "cure" schizophrenia, but only facilitate remissions of the disease. It is a very sad but probably true statement, at least for most of these patients, that "once a schizophrenic, always a schizophrenic." Despite this caveat, we still should feel heartened that the blockade of dopamine receptors is indeed the most meaningful action of phenothiazines as far as schizophrenia is concerned. Moreover, research related to the mechanism of action of amphetamines further bolsters the hypothesis that dopamine and schizophrenia have something important to do with each other.

How Amphetamines Act

In trying to understand the actions of amphetamines, pharmacologists have a headstart over other drugs; for there are extremely close chemical similarities between amphetamine and norepinephrine and dopamine. Thus, it has long been an article of faith among pharmacologists that, one way or another, amphetamines exert their therapeutic actions via norepinephrine and/or dopamine. Direct experimentation has revealed a number of ways in which amphetamines can interact with norepinephrine and dopamine.

Two actions appear to be responsible for the therapeutic and not-so-therapeutic effects of the amphetamines. Amphetamine can directly release norepinephrine or dopamine into the synaptic cleft. Amphetamine is also quite effective in blocking the re-uptake mechanism whereby norepinephrine and dopamine are normally inactivated. Such a blockade of the re-uptake process would result in more norepinephrine or dopamine piling up within the synaptic cleft. In this way, amphetamine can potentiate the actions of norepinephrine or dopamine normally released by nerves firing. The relative role played by amphetamine's ability to release norepinephrine and dopamine and its ability to block the re-uptake is not all together clear. Indeed, it is possible that the releasing action of amphetamine and its blockade of re-uptake are closely related processes which are mutually interdependent, so that they cannot be separated. In any event, by either mechanism one would obtain more norepinephrine and dopamine in the synaptic cleft and, hence, a facilitation of whatever the usual actions are of norepinephrine and dopamine when released by neurons.

The interactions of cocaine with brain norepinephrine and dopamine are not as well worked out as those with amphetamine. However, it is well established that cocaine can block the re-uptake inactivation of norepinephrine and dopamine, an effect which it would thus share with amphetamines. In this way cocaine would be able to facilitate norepinephrine and dopamine effects just as does amphetamine. Whether cocaine has a releasing action on norepinephrine and dopamine as well has not yet been established.

Just by making use of the little bit of information we have about the various norepinephrine and dopamine pathways in the brain, we can make some fairly educated guesses about which of the tracts mediates particular behavioral actions of amphetamines. For instance, most people agree that the cerebral cortex is the organ most responsible for "higher" mental function, which demand alertness as well as careful intellectual and sensory discrimination. Perhaps the ability of amphetamine and cocaine to facilitate intellectual performance is mediated by fibers of the dorsal norepinephrine pathway passing to the cerebral cortex.

As we mentioned before, the cerebellum is responsible for fine coordination of muscular movements. Perhaps the norepinephrine tracts passing to this part of the brain are responsible for the ability of amphetamine and cocaine to facilitate the performance of subtle and complex motor tasks. It would be reasonable to speculate that any effect of amphetamine on the fibers of the ventral norepinephrine pathway which enter the "pleasure centers" in the hypothalamus may account for the euphoria evoked by amphetamine and cocaine.

CATECHOLAMINES AND AMPHETAMINE PSYCHOSIS

What about amphetamine psychosis? Which of the two, dopamine or norepinephrine, might be related to this important "model schizophrenia?" Of course, to our knowledge there is no valid animal model of psychosis. Ideally, one would like to devise an experimental approach in humans to answer this question. As we discussed in the chapter on stimulants, drugs often exist in mirror-image forms. Dextroamphetamine, the form which rotates light to the right, is about five times more potent a central stimulant in man than is levoamphetamine, which rotates light to the left. Studies in our own laboratory as well as those of Drs. Burton Angrist in

New York and John Davis at Vanderbilt University have utilized these mirror-image differences to shed light on the relative roles of dopamine and norepinephrine in mediating behavioral effects of amphetamines. While technical problems make interpretations difficult, it appears that amphetamine psychosis and the exacerbation of schizophrenic symptoms by amphetaminelike drugs may primarily involve brain dopamine. By contrast norepinephrine seems most responsible for the central stimulant alerting effects of amphetamine.

Earlier, we asked why amphetamine invariably elicited paranoid psychoses rather than some other form of schizophrenialike psychosis. We suggested that the ability of amphetamine to cause psychosis and its central stimulant actions might be quite distinct. Amphetamine could provoke a schizophrenialike picture whose paranoid flavor was conferred by the central stimulant actions of the drug.

The experimental results with amphetamine isomers just described suggest that the psychosis elicited by amphetamine may be mediated by brain dopamine. By contrast, one would expect central stimulant actions of amphetamine to be mediated by brain norepinephrine. One might speculate, therefore, that the norepine-phrine-mediated alerting action represents that effect of amphetamine which converts the schizophrenialike psychosis into a paranoid one. How might the alerting action of amphetamine, mediated by norepinephrine, convert the schizophrenialike picture into a paranoid psychosis? As discussed earlier, the alerting action might force the patient to strive for an intellectual way in which to explain all his strange alterations in his sense of self. By its norepinephrine mediated alerting effects, the schizophrenialike picture would be converted into a paranoid psychosis. Thus a "schizophrenialike" component of amphetamine psychosis may be mediated primarily by brain dopamine, while the "paranoid solution" is facilitated by the drug's alerting actions via stimulation of norepinephrine systems.

And if indeed the norepinephrine-mediated alerting actions of amphetamines interact with and "contaminate" a purer dopamine-mediated amphetamine psychosis, then removal of these "norepinephrine effects" might leave one with an amphetamine psychosis more closely resembling schizophrenia then the present version. Conceivably a drug that would stimulate dopamine but not norepinephrine mechanisms in the brain would produce a more "pure" model of schizophrenia. Though these nations are tantalizing and provocative, please remember that they are unproven, tentative speculations.

Tying It All Together

In talking about schizophrenia we had speculated that the primary disorder might lie in the inability to integrate perceptions in a "sane" fashion with internal feelings and memories. Neurophysiologic studies of how the phenothiazines act had suggested that they might "ward off" the onslaught of intolerable perceptions. The notion was that this warding off was not equivalent to simply diminishing sensory input so that whoever took the drug would be to a certain extent deaf and blind. Instead, phenothiazines presumably diminished the ability of perceptions to impinge upon internal mental states of the patient in the "crazy" way which they have been doing in the schizophrenic. Now we have suggested that phenothiazines act by blocking certain unspecified dopamine systems in the brain and that amphetamines and cocaine activate the same systems. Is there any evidence that the dopamine neurons in the brain might have anything to do with integrating sensory perception and internal states of the mind?

Until one or two years ago it was widely thought that the only definite function of dopamine neurons, especially the system connecting the substantia nigra and corpus striatum, had to do with coordinating bodily movements. Then, as described above, Dr. Urban Ungerstedt discovered that this same set of dopamine neurons was intimately tied up with the control of eating and drinking. More recently, Ungerstedt has found further functions for this dopamine system.

When he destroyed the dopamine neurons connecting the substantia nigra and the corpus striatum on one side of the brain, he found that rats ceased to pay attention at all to sensory stimulation presented to the other side of their bodies. They would pay no heed to touching, pinching, smells, or visual stimuli presented to the side opposite to that on which the dopamine neurons had been destroyed. This "sensory neglect" did not represent an absence of sensory perception. In other words, these animals were not blind, deaf, and unable to feel on one side of their bodies. By a variety of experimental procedures, Ungerstedt showed that sensation itself was intact. Rather, the animals simply did not pay any attention to things that they perceived. Ungerstedt feels that these animals have lost the ability to integrate their perceptions with their internal memories and feelings and therefore cannot motivate themselves to respond to their perceptions. He feels that the same thing is going on when rats refuse to eat or drink after destruction of the dopamine systems on both sides of the brain. They perceive the food and water but cannot "act" to alleviate their hunger and thirst.

One can readily conceptualize the way Ungerstedt's recent discoveries could mesh well with the thoughts we have been presenting regarding phenothiazines and amphetamines. Since the "world is too much" for schizophrenics, phenothiazines might help them to cope by blocking dopamine receptors, thus decreasing the activity of dopamine systems and thereby divorcing sensory perceptions from the internal feelings and memories upon which they normally impinge. All of this would make the environment more bearable without causing true sensory deprivation or acting as a sedative and virtually putting the patient to sleep. Amphetamines, however, stimulate these dopamine systems, thereby exposing the internal states of the patient to his noxious environment more than ever before. In massive doses administered constantly for days at a time, one can see how this would make even a normal person psychotic. With the schizophrenic, who is already in a tenuous equilibrium, even small doses would be enough to exacerbate his illness.

Again we must wonder exactly which dopamine systems could be responsible for this grand scheme. Most of Ungerstedt's research was directed at the major dopamine tract connecting the substantia nigra and corpus striatum—though when he destroyed this tract he, at the same time, injured other dopamine pathways—to the nucleus accumbens and olfactory tubercle. If this were the sole tract involved, one would expect to find more remarkable psychological changes in patients with Parkinson's disease then is usually reported. On the other hand, perhaps one would not anticipate any remarkable psychological alterations. One might even predict that the only unique psychological feature of patients with Parkinson's disease would be that they would be relatively resistant to schizophrenic breakdown. To my knowledge no one has studied the exact frequency of schizophrenia in patients with Parkinson's disease or whether schizophrenics who develop Parkinson's disease improve. An important item to bear in mind is that Ungerstedt's research in rats may not apply directly to humans. Although many facts about the relationship of dopamine and drugs in rats fit in nicely with clinical observations in humans, it is quite conceivable that specific dopamine tracts responsible for particular behaviors might differ in humans and animals. And as mentioned above, Ungerstedt's operative procedures affected several dopamine tracts in the rat besides the one related to Parkinson's disease.

Final Words of Caution and Hope

All of what we have discussed in this chapter suggests that drugs relevant to schizophrenia interact in an important way with dopamine systems in the brain. What is particularly nice is the possibility that this biochemical information may fit in smoothly with what we know about the psychology of schizophrenia and psychological and neurophysiological mechanisms, by which drugs relieve the symptoms of schizophrenia. It would be most pleasant at this stage to conclude that all of this is telling us something about the primary disorder in the brains of schizophrenic patients. But, as I have emphasized many times already, when we get to this level of speculation we must tread lightly. No specific biochemical abnormality has ever been demonstrated in the body fluids or brains of schizophrenics. The rich body of information we have been reviewing certainly sheds much light on how drugs relevant to schizophrenia exert their effects in the brain. There is a good chance that amphetamines do indeed elicit psychosis via dopamine systems and that phenothiazines relieve the symptoms of schizophrenia and of amphetamine psychosis by altering the same systems.

Some of the psychological functions of the dopamine neuron remind us of what seems to be psychologically wrong in schizophrenics. But reminding and knowing are not the same thing. Here we are grasping at what is unknown. When one grasps at the unknown, his chances of being right are certainly small. But the attempt makes us think hard and search still harder. And I know of no other course.

Appendix I

Neurotransmitters

In the text of the book we talked exclusively about the catecholamines, norepinephrine, and dopamine as neurotransmitters. Although these compounds are of great importance In regulating emotional behavior, they are not the major transmitters in the brain. In the hypothalamus, where norepinephrine occurs in higher concentrations than anyplace else in the brain, only about five percent of the nerve endings contain norepinephrine. And in the corpus striatum, where dopamine is the major catecholamine and more dopamine exists then anywhere else in the brain, only fifteen percent of the nerve endings contain dopamine. There are numerous other major neurotransmitters which we will consider.

CATECHOLAMINES

First, let us describe a little of the chemistry of the catecholamines. As depicted in Figure 1 the chemical

HISTAMINE

$(CH_3)_3-N-CH_2-CH_2-O-\underset{\underset{O}{\|}}{C}-CH_3$

ACETYLCHOLINE

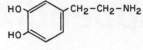

DOPAMINE

$H_2N-CH_2-CH_2-CH_2-COOH$

GABA (Gamma–Aminobutyric Acid)

NOREPINEPHRINE

H_2N-CH_2-COOH

GLYCINE

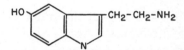

SEROTONIN (5-Hydroxytryptamine)

$HOOC-CH_2-CH_2-\underset{\underset{NH_2}{|}}{CH}-COOH$

GLUTAMIC ACID

FIGURE 1

structures of norepinephrine and dopamine are quite similar. They are called catecholamines, because the benzene ring (the hexagon with the internal lines) contains two adjacent hydroxyl groupings (a hydroxyl is an oxygen attached to a hydrogen). The definition of "catechol" is a benzene ring with two adjacent hydroxyl groups. The amine part of the molecule refers to the nitrogen of the side chain. All known neurotransmitters have amine groups which appear to key parts of the molecule for interacting with the receptor.

Dopamine differs from norepinephrine only in the absence of a hydroxyl group on the side chain at the beta carbon (one counts the carbons of the side chain beginning with the amine grouping, so that the carbon attached directly to the amine is called the alpha carbon and the next one the beta carbon).

How are catecholamines formed in the body? Almost all neurotransmitters seem to originate as products of amino acids. Amino acids contain both acid groupings called "carboxyl" groups and amine groups. Amino acids are best known as the building blocks of proteins. There are about twenty major naturally occurring amino acids which are linked together in varying sequences to provide all the hundreds of thousands of proteins that the body normally can make. However, amino acids have many other functions besides entering into proteins. From our point of view, they are crucial as the precursors of neurotransmitters.

Tyrosine is the amino acid precursor of the catecholamines. As is evident in Figure 2, tyrosine contains only one hydroxyl group on the benzene ring. An enzyme, tyrosine hydroxylase, adds another hydroxyl group so that the product is now a catechol. (Enzymes are proteins which catalyze the majority of chemical reactions in the body.) The product of tyrosine hydroxylase activity is dihydroxyphenylalanine, which is referred to as "dopa" for short. Like many other chemicals in the body, dopa can exist as one of two mirror image forms. The naturally occurring form is designated L-dopa. The body will not make use of D-dopa for conversion to catecholamines, so that if one wants to utilize dopa as a precursor of catecholamines, it is best to administer L-dopa.

The carboxyl group is removed from dopa via an

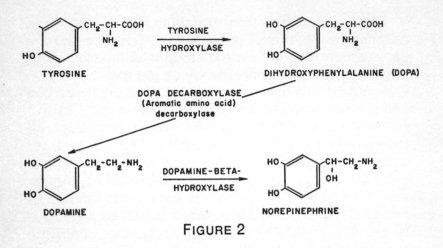

FIGURE 2

enzyme called dopa decarboxylase which results in the formation of dopamine. Dopamine is transformed to norepinephrine within norepinephrine neurons by an enzyme which adds on the hydroxyl group at the beta position. This enzyme is therefore called dopamine beta hydroxylase. Thus dopamine has two jobs. In norepinephrine neurons, it is *not* a neurotransmitter but only the precursor of the neurotransmitter, norepinephrine. Dopamine neurons contain neither norepinephrine nor the enzyme to transform dopamine into norepinephrine, so that here dopamine acts as the neurotransmitter.

Mirror image chemistry, or stereochemistry, has played a key role in some of our discussions. What determines whether a chemical will have "different" mirror image forms is simply whether or not it is asymmetrical.

When viewed in a mirror a symetrical structure is not altered, but an asymetrical one is indeed different. One can have right-handed and left-handed baseball mitts, but there is only one "steric" class of tennis racquets.

Since the basic skeleton of most chemicals in the body is formed by carbon atoms, the asymmetry lies among the carbons. Carbon atoms can be linked chemically with as many as four other atoms. A given carbon atom in a molecule is asymmetric only when all four links are to four different types of atoms. Dopamine is not asymmetric, because every one of its carbons contain more than one linkage of the same sort. For instance, look at the beta carbon of dopamine. It contains two hydrogens which, of course, are identical so that the beta position is not asymmetric. Therefore dopamine, like the tennis racquet, does not exist in different mirror image forms. By contrast, substitution of one of those hydrogens by a hydroxyl group transforms dopamine into norepinephrine which now is asymmetric at the beta position. Therefore, there can be two mirror image forms of norepinephrine. The one which rotates a plane of polarized light to the left is called levo- or l-norepinephrine and the other is dextro- or d-norepinephrine. The naturally occurring form is l-norepinephrine.

SEROTONIN

Serotonin, which is also called 5-hydroxytryptamine, is made in the body from the amino acid tryptophan. Serotonin occurs in even fewer neurons than does norepinephrine or dopamine. Like norepinephrine the highest concentrations of serotonin are in the hypothalamus. The same Swedish researchers who developed the fluorescent stain for catecholamines found that their stain worked quite nicely in revealing the localization of serotonin neurons. While norepinephrine and dopamine fluoresce bright green in the presence of formaldehyde, serotonin fluoresces bright yellow. Thus it is quite easy to distinguish between serotonin and the catecholamines. The serotonin neuronal pathways in the brain have been mapped out just as have those of the catecholamines. The cell bodies for the serotonin neurons are all clustered in the midline of the brain stem, in a grouping known as the "raphe" series of nuclei. The raphe nuclei were know to anatomists long before the Swedish researchers identified serotonin within cells of the raphe nuclei. Now it is known that the raphe nuclei contain exclusively serotonin cells. Axons from these cells ascend and give off nerve endings throughout the brain.

The functions of serotonin neurons are less well understood then are those of the catecholamines. However, it is reasonably certain that serotonin neurons play some role in regulating sleep and wakefulness. If serotonin neurons are selectively destroyed in such a fashion that the brain is depleted by ninety percent of its serotonin content, animals will become insomniac for prolonged periods. Depleting serotonin from the brain by treatment with drugs which block its formation also causes insomnia. Interestingly, animals who have been rendered insomniac by brain lesions or blockade of serotonin synthesis can be put to sleep by a simple injection of the amino acid precursor of serotonin.

HISTAMINE

Histamine concentrations in the brain are only about a tenth those of norepinephrine and serotonin. If the concentration of a neurotransmitter in the brain reflects the number of neurons in which it serves as a transmitter (a rule to which there are probably many exceptions), one would suspect that histamine is not a transmitter at a large number of synapses. There are no techniques to visualize histamine under the microscope. However, by other technical procedures it has been possible to show that histamine is highly localized to nerve endings in the brain and therefore is probably a neurotransmitter. Interestingly, like norepinephrine and serotonin, histamine is also highly concentrated in the hypothalamus, which perhaps should provide some hints as to its normal function.

Acetylcholine is the oldest of the neurotransmitters in terms of its scientific recognition. Acetylcholine is definitely established as the neurotransmitter at the neuromuscular junction (that is to say, the point of linkup between nerves and the voluntary muscles of the body). Voluntary muscles are those which we can move of our own volition, such as the muscles of our face, arms, and legs. By contrast, involuntary muscles are those of the heart and intestines and other organs which contract and relax outside of normal human awareness. Acetylcholine is also the transmitter to certain of these involuntary muscles and in a major portion of the entire "involuntary" nervous system outside of the brain.

The portion of the "involuntary" nervous system in which acetylcholine is a transmitter is called the "parasympathetic" system. The types of effects which are obtained when one stimulates the parasympathetic nervous system are slowing of the heart, constriction of the pupils of the eyes, and contraction of the intestines. These are the sorts of functions associated with everyday, nonemergency behavior.

By contrast, the sympathetic nervous system is a portion of the involuntary nervous system which regulates emergency, "fight-or-flight" behavior. When the sympathetic nervous system fires, the heart speeds up; blood vessels constrict to elevate blood pressure; the pupils dilate, presumably to allow one to view the dangers in the environment more clearly; and the bronchial tubes dilate, to make heavy breathing proceed more readily. The principal neurotransmitter of the sympathetic nervous system is norepinephrine. It is quite interesting that the sympathetic nervous system outside the brain in which norepinephrine serves as a transmitter is concerned with excitation and general alerting behavior. Similarly, within the brain, as we discussed within the text of the book, the firing of norepinephrine neurons seems to provoke an excited, euphoric state.

AMINO ACID NEUROTRANSMITTERS

The major neurotransmitters, at least those which account for communication at the largest number of synapses, appear to be amino acids. One of the best known of these is gamma-aminobutyric acid, usually referred to simply as GABA. GABA appears to be a neurotransmitter in anywhere between thirty and fifty percent of the synapses within the brain. When applied directly to neurons, it invariably slows their firing rates, hence is said to be an "inhibitory" neurotransmitter. Since GABA acts at so many synapses in the brain and is inhibitory, one would expect that a blockade of GABA effects would cause the reverse of inhibition, namely, overexcitation. Indeed, bicuculline, a drug which blocks GABA receptors, cause convulsions.

Like the catecholamines, GABA is inactivated by re-uptake into the nerves which had released it. If one had a drug which blocked GABA re-uptake efficiently, such a drug might increase inhibition throughout the nervous system and therefore be a useful anticonvulsant drug. At the present time (1973) there is no potent and general effective inhibitor of GABA uptake.

GABA has no other function, to our knowledge, except to serve as a neurotransmitter. By contrast, glycine is an amino acid which serves as a constituent of proteins and has a variety of functions in the total metabolic scheme of the body. But glycine also appears to be a major inhibitory transmitter, especially in the spinal cord and brain stem. Strychnine, a well-known convulsant drug, is a very specific blocker of glycine receptors.

If glycine and GABA are the major inhibitory neurotransmitters one might expect there to be one or more major excitatory neurotransmitters. Definitive evidence is not yet available for the existence of the "universal excitatory neurotransmitter." However, there is a lot of circumstantial evidence suggesting that glutamic acid, another amino acid, may serve such a role in the brain. Like glycine, glutamic acid is a component of many proteins and has a variety of general metabolic functions. The brain contains a great deal of glutamic acid, in fact more than any other amino acid. Concentrations of glutamic acid in the brain are about a thousand times greater than those of norepinephrine, dopamine, and serotonin. Because glutamic acid serves so many other functions in the brain, it is hard to explore its neurotransmitter role in a rigorous fashion. Unfortunately, unlike the situation with glycine and GABA, there are no specific blockers of glutamic acid effects. Thus the task of determining the precise function of glutamic acid in the brain is quite difficult.

Appendix II

Psychotropic Drugs

AMPHETAMINE AND RELATED DRUGS

When one compares the structure of amphetamine depicted in Figure 1 with that of the catecholamines in the preceding appendix, it is evident why pharmacologists have always felt secure in assuming that amphetamines act via one or another of the catecholamines in the brain. Note how the alpha carbon of amphetamine is linked to four distinct atoms so that amphetamine is asymmetric at the alpha carbon. Methamphetamine differs from amphetamine only in the addition of a methyl group on the amine. Methylphenidate, whose trade name is Ritalin, is an amphetamine derivative with little appetite-suppressing effect but which is a potent central stimulant. On the other hand, phenmetrazine, or Preludin, is supposed to have more appetite-suppress-

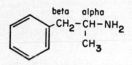

AMPHETAMINE

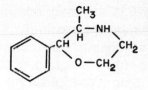

PHENMETRAZINE (Preludin)

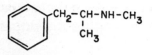

METHAMPHETAMINE (Methedrine)

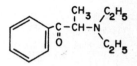

DIETHYLPROPION (Tenuate)

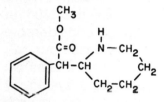

METHYLPHENIDATE (Ritalin)

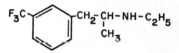

FENFLURAMINE

FIGURE 1

ing than stimulant effects. The same is said to be true for diethylpropion (Tenuate). However, as attested by the great Preludin epidemic in Sweden, it is likely that the animal evidence regarding the relative amount of central stimulant activity of amphetamine analogues doesn't apply in a meaningful fashion to man.

Fenfluramine is a drug related to the amphetamines which effectively suppresses appetite but which is truly not a central stimulant. In fact, it tends to sedate users. Fenfluramine should be the ideal appetite-suppressing drug. It has been marketed in Europe but has not yet

(1973) attained commercial application in the United States. Interestingly, I have heard that fenfluramine is not selling particularly well in Europe. At a recent scientific meeting, pharmacologists were informally discussing this puzzling situation. Some of them speculated that what the plump housewives seek when they use amphetamine is not so much appetite suppression but mood elevation. This euphoria in turn provides the sense of vitality that enables them to endure the rigors of dieting.

ANTISCHIZOPHRENIC DRUGS

Thousands upon thousands of phenothiazines have been synthesized over the years. Those depicted in Figure 2 are the ones which have gained considerable utility. The phenothiazine drugs do not resemble catecholamines in an obvious way as do amphetamines. Their three rings linked together provide a system of resonating electrons which are highly reactive chemically. These electrons, which hover in a cloud about the ring system, are responsible for many of the multiple biochemical effects of the phenothiazines.

The phenothiazine drugs can be grouped into at least two classes, depending on the structure of their side chains. One group, whose side chains might be referred to as "alkylamino," tend to produce more sedating side effects as well as to lower blood pressure. The alkylamino phenothiazine drugs are also less potent on a weight basis than the other drugs. Chlorpromazine is the classic example of the alkylamino group.

The phenothiazine drugs which contain piperazine rings in their side chains are referred to as the "piperazine" phenothiazine drugs. They act in smaller doses and produce less sedation and lowering of blood pres-

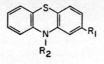

Phenothiazine nucleus

	R_1	R_2
		ALKYLAMINO
Chlorpromazine (Thorazine)	Cl	$CH_2-CH_2-CH_2-N-(CH_3)_2$
Promazine (Sparine)	—	$CH_2-CH_2-CH_2-N-(CH_3)_2$
Triflupromazine (Vesprin)	CF_3	$CH_2-CH_2-CH_2-N-(CH_3)_2$
		PIPERAZINE
Prochlorperazine (Compazine)	Cl	$CH_2-CH_2-CH_2-N\diagdown\diagup N-CH_3$
Trifluoperazine (Stelazine)	CF_3	$CH_2-CH_2-CH_2-N\diagdown\diagup N-CH_3$
Perphenazine (Trilafon)	Cl	$CH_2-CH_2-CH_2-N\diagdown\diagup N-CH_2-CH_2-OH$
Fluphenazine (Prolixin; Permitil)	CF_3	$CH_2-CH_2-CH_2-N\diagdown\diagup N-CH_2-CH_2-OH$
Thiopropazate (Dartal)	Cl	$CH_2-CH_2-CH_2-N\diagdown\diagup N-CH_2-CH_2-O\overset{O}{\overset{\|}{C}}-CH_3$
		PIPERIDINE
Thioridazine (Mellaril)	SCH_3	$CH_2-CH_2-CH\diagdown$ (N-methyl piperidine ring)
Mepazine (Pacatal)	—	(N-methyl piperidine ring)

FIGURE 2

sure than do the alkylamino phenothiazines. However, these drugs produce a much higher incidence of Parkinsonian-like side effects than do the alkylamino phenothiazines. In treating patients, psychiatrists usually start with a drug from one class and, if side effects are intolerable, switch to the other class. Thioridazine (Mellaril) has a "ring" in its side chain which, however, is not a piperazine ring. So it is neither alkylamino nor piperazine. Thioridazine, which is one of the most widely used phenothiazines, behaves in patients essentially like the alkylamino phenothiazines.

The Parkinsonian-like side effects of the phenothiazine drugs are more properly called "extra-pyramidal" side effects since they are not exactly like Parkinson's disease. The word "extra-pyramidal" refers to a general class of body movements. There are a number of different extra-pyramidal side effects. One consists of symptoms mimicking closely those of a patient with Parkinson's disease. These include rigidity of all the muscles of the face and extremities and a coarse tremor of the extremities. Besides Parkinsonian-like symptoms, patients may develop strange muscular contortions, such as a twisting of the head to the side, rolling of the eyes back in their sockets, and a profuse production of saliva which dribbles out of the mouth. Perhaps the most interesting extra-pyramidal side effect of the phenothiazine drugs is called "akathisia." Akathisia refers to a funny feeling of muscular "itchiness." Patients are unable to sit still and feel obliged to pace up and down the floor. Unfortunately, inexperienced hospital staff often assume that the patient is becoming quite agitated and "treat" this disturbance by increasing doses of the phenothiazines, creating a vicious cycle.

The butyrophenones differ greatly in their chemical structure from the phenothiazine drugs. However, for some inexplicable reason, their pharmacological actions are virtually identical to those of the phenothiazines. They tend to behave like the piperazine side chain phenothiazines in their spectrum of actions. Thus the butyrophenone drugs are the most potent of all the antischizophrenic drugs, some acting in doses as little as one one-thousandth of the typical therapeutic dose of chlorpromazine. The butyrophenones, however, produce the highest incidence of extra-pyramidal side effects. In some studies, almost every patient manifested some extra-pyramidal side effects with anti-Parkinsonian drugs.

Part of the initial difficulty in securing general acceptance to the hypothesis that dopamine receptor blockade explains the clinical actions of the phenothiazines was the lack of chemical similarity between phenothiazines and catecholamines. Most phenothiazines are complex multi-ringed structures, while dopamine is a simple phenylethylamine. Recently Alan Horn and I reexamined this question. We studied the conformation, or shape, of the chlorpromazine molecule which other scientists had determined by the technique of X-ray crystallography. We noticed that chlorpromazine, in this "optimal" shape, would be quite capable of mimicking the dopamine molecule at its receptor sites.

In the preferred conformation of chlorpromazine, its side chain tilts away from the midline toward the chlorine-substituted ring (Figure 3). Presumably the chlorine on Ring A is responsible for the "tilt" of the side chain, since, if there were no substituent on Ring A, both Rings A and C would be symmetrical and one

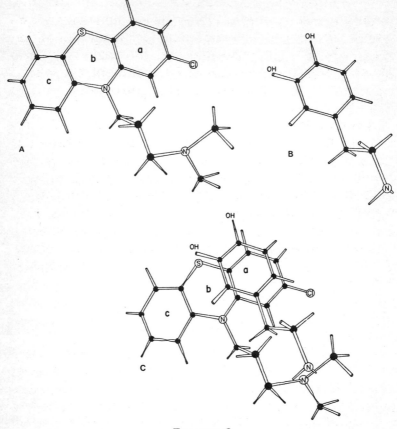

FIGURE 3

would expect the side chain to be fully extended, that is, to stick straight out halfway in between Rings A and C, rather than tilting toward one or the other. Accordingly, phenothiazine drugs lacking a substituent on Ring A should be less capable of mimicking the conformation of dopamine, and therefore have less affinity for dopamine receptors and presumably be less effective in the treatment of schizophrenia. Of a dozen or so phenothiazine tranquilizers which have been widely employed clinically, only two of them lack a substituent on Ring A. Strikingly, mepazine and promazine, the two phenothiazines lacking a Ring A substituent, are indeed significantly less effective as antischizophrenic drugs than the others.

Besides the Ring A substituent, another major requirement for therapeutic activity of phenothiazines is separation of the side chain amine by three carbon atoms from the ring system. Molecular models indicate that shortening the side chain to two carbon atoms would make the assumption of the dopaminelike conformation less likely. Just as predicted, phenothiazines with two carbon side chains, such as the antihistamine promethazine, lack therapeutic effectiveness in schizophrenia.

ANTIDEPRESSANT DRUGS

The principal antidepressant drugs used in psychiatry are referred to as a group as the "tricyclic" antidepressants, because they have a three-ring system much like the phenothiazine drugs. Indeed these compounds were developed as potential antischizophrenic drugs. An astute Swiss psychiatrist recognized that they were capable of relieving depression in some patients. Because of the close relationship between phenothiazines and the tricyclic antidepressants, some of the phenothiazines have been given to depressed patients and found to be useful drugs. However, the tricyclic antidepressants are not at all effective in schizophrenia.

How do the tricyclic antidepressants act? These compounds are highly potent in blocking the re-uptake process of norepinephrine neurons. Since re-uptake of norepinephrine by the nerve endings which have released it accounts for its inactivation at synapses, the antidepressant drugs thus facilitate the synaptic activities of norepinephrine. In this way they share one of the actions of amphetamines.

Antidepressant drugs rarely produce euphoria directly. Rather, over a period of ten days to two weeks there is a gradual relief of the depression. Why don't the antidepressants and amphetamines produce the same clinical effects? Amphetamine itself makes depressed patients euphoric, but when administered for a prolonged period it is not effective in relieving their depression.

One explanation for this discrepancy may have to do with the time course of action of these drugs. The tricyclic antidepressants do not seem to accumulate in the blood and brain very rapidly, so that a week or more is required for them to reach therapeutic levels. Perhaps, for adequate relief of depression, one wishes to develop the potentiation of norepinephrine gradually. By contrast, amphetamine exerts its effects quite rapidly. Conceivably this "rapid-fire" euphoric stimulation jars the equilibrium of the depressed patient and thus may even tend to make him worse.

Another possibility for a difference between the tricyclic antidepressants and amphetamines has to do with interactions with other neurotransmitters. Amphetamine itself has few effects upon brain serotonin. Serotonin is inactivated by a re-uptake system into the nerve endings of serotonin neurons, analogous to the norepinephrine re-uptake system. Most tricyclic antidepressants are just as potent in blocking serotonin re-uptake as they are in blocking norepinephrine re-uptake. Therefore, a number of scientists have hypothesized that these drugs relieve depression by potentiating serotonin as well as norepinephrine.

Amphetamine does not potentiate serotonin by blocking its re-uptake as do the tricyclic antidepressants. If potentiation of serotonin is important for the relief of depression, one would accordingly not expect amphetamine to be a powerful antidepressant.

References

Chapter 1

Rosenhan, D. L. "On Being Sane in Insane Places." *Science,* Vol. 197, No. 4070, pp. 250–258, 1973.

Chapter 2

Bradley, P. B., and Key, B. J. "The Effect of Drugs on Arousal Responses Produced by Electrical Stimulation of the Reticular Formation of the Brain." *Electroencephalog. Clin. Neurophysiol.,* Vol. 10, p. 97, 1958.

Casey, J. F., Bennett, I. F., Lindley, C. J., Hollister, L. E., Gordon, M. H., and Springer, N. N. "Drug Therapy and Schizophrenia. A Controlled Study of the Effectiveness of Chlorpromazine, Promazine, Phenobarbital and Placebo." *Archives of General Psychiatry,* Vol. 2, pp. 210–220, 1960.

———, Lasky, J. J., Klett, C. J., and Hollister, L. E. "Treatment of Schizophrenic Reactions with Phenothiazine Derivatives. A Comparative Study of Chlorpromazine, Triflupromazine, Mepazine, Prochlorperazine, Perphenazine and Phenobarbital." *American Journal of Psychiatry,* Vol. 117, pp. 97–105, 1960.

Chapman, C. J., and Knowles, R. R. "The Effects of Phenothiazines on Disordered Thought in Schizophrenia." *Journal of Consulting Psychology,* Vol. 28, pp. 165–169, 1964.

Cole, J. O. "Phenothiazine Treatment in Acute Schizophrenia." *Archives of General Psychiatry,* Vol. 10, pp. 246–261, 1964.

Davis, J. M. "The Efficacy of the Tranquillizing and Antidepressant Drugs." *Archives of General Psychiatry,* Vol. 13, pp. 552–572, 1965.

Delay, J., and Deniker, P. "Le Traitement des psychoses par une methode neurolytique derivée d'hibernothérapie; le 4560 RP utilisée seul en cure prolongée et continuée." *C. R. Congr. Alién. Neurol. France,* Vol. 50, pp. 497–502, 1952.

————, and Deniker, P. "38 cas des psychoses traitées par la cure prolongée et continuée de 4560 RP." *C. R. Congr. Alién Neurol. France,* Vol. 50. pp. 503–513, 1952.

Deniker, P. "Introduction of Neuroleptic Chemotherapy into Psychiatry." In *Discoveries in Biological Psychiatry,* F. J. Ayd and B. Blackwell, editors, Lippincott, Philadelphia, pp. 155–164 (1970).

Dimascio, A., Havens, L. L., and Klerman, G. L. "The Psychopharmacology of Phenothiazine Compounds: A Comparative Study of the Effects of Chlorpromazine, Promethazine, Trifluoperazine, and Perphenazine in Normal Males. II: Results and Discussion." *Journal of Nervous and Mental Diseases,* Vol. 136, pp. 168–186, 1963.

Gorham, D. R., and Pokorny, A. D. "Effects of a Phenothiazine and/or Group Psychotherapy with Schizophrenics," *Diseases of the Nervous System,* Vol. 25, pp. 77–86, 1964.

Klein, D. S., and Davis, J. M. "Diagnosis and Drug Treatment of Psychiatric Disorders." Williams and Wilkins Company, Baltimore (1969).

Kurland, A. A., Michaux, M. H., Hanlon, T. E., Ota, K. Y., and Simopoulos, A. M. "The Comparative Effectiveness of Six Phenothiazine Compounds, Phenobarbital and Inert Placebo in the Treatment of Acutely Ill Patients: Personality Dimensions." *Journal of Nervous and Mental Diseases,* Vol. 134, pp. 48–61, 1962.

Laborit, H. "La thérapeutique neuro-végétate du choc et de la maladie post-traumatique." *Presse Medicale,* Vol. 58, pp. 138–140, 1950.

————, Huguenard, P., and Alluaume, R. "Un nouveau stabilisateur végétatif (le 4560 RP)." *Presse Medicale,* Vol. 60, pp. 206–208, 1952.

Moore, R. B., Pierce, W. J., and Dennison, A. D., Jr. "The Story of Reserpine." *Journal of the Indiana State Medical Association,* Vol. 47, p. 854, 1954.

Muller, J. M., Schlittler, E., and Bein, H. J. *Experientia,* Vol. 8, p. 338, 1952.

National Institute of Mental Health–Psychopharmacology Service Center Collaborative Study Group. "Phenothiazine Treatment in Acute Schizophrenia: Effectiveness." *Archives of General Psychiatry,* Vol. 10, pp. 246–261, 1964.

Noce, Williams, and Rappaport, cited by Pfieffer, C. C., and Murphree, H. B., in *Pharmacology in Medicine,* J. R. Dipalma, editor. McGraw-Hill Book Company, New York, p. 321 (1965).

Ray, O. S. *Drugs, Society and Human Behavior,* C. V. Mosby Company, St. Louis, p. 143 (1972).

Zebulun Column "Serendipity," *Arch. Int. Med.,* Vol. 111, pp. 385–386, 1963.

Chapter 3

Anonymous, "An Autobiography of a Schizophrenic Experience." *J. Abnorm. Soc. Psychol.,* Vol. 51, pp. 677–689, 1955.

Blacker, K. H., Jones, R. T., Stone, G. C., and Pfefferbaum, D. "Chronic Users of LSD: The Acidheads." *Amer. J. Psychiat.,* Vol. 125, pp. 341–351, 1968.

Bowers, M. B., Jr., and Freedman, D. X. "Psychedelic Experiences in Acute Psychosis." *Arch. Gen. Psychiat.,* Vol. 15, pp. 240–248, 1966.

Feinberg, I. "A Comparison of the Visual Hallucinations in Schizophrenia with Those Induced by Mescaline and LSD-25." In *Hallucinations,* L. J. West, editor. Grune and Stratton, New York, pp. 64–76 (1962).

Gautier, T. *The Hashish Club.* Harper and Row, New York, p. 41, (1971).

Hoffer. A., Osmond, H., and Smythies, J. R. "Schizophrenia: A New Approach." *J. Ment. Sci.,* Vol. 100, pp. 29–45, 1954.

Hollister, L. E. "Drug-Induced Psychoses and Schizophrenic Reactions: A Critical Comparison." *Ann. N. Y. Acad. Sci.,* Vol. 96, pp. 80–88, 1962.

Houston, J. "Phenomenology of the Psychedelic Experience." In *Psychedelic Drugs,* R. E. Hicks and P. J. Fink, editors. Grune and Stratton, New York, pp. 1–7 (1969).

Huxley, A. *The Doors of Perception.* Harper and Row, New York (1954).

Jaspers, K. *General Psychopathology.* Manchester University Press, Manchester, pp. 417–418 (1962).

Kast, E. C., and Collins, V. J. "A Study of Lysergic Acid Diethylamide as an Analgesic Agent." *Anesthesia, and Analgesia,* Vol. 43, pp. 285–291 (1964).

Kurland, A. A., Unger, S. M., Schaffer, J. W., and Savage, C. "Psychedelic Therapy Utilizing LSD in the Treatment of the Alcoholic Patient: A Preliminary Report." *Am. J. Psychiat.,* Vol. 123, pp. 1202, 1967.

Laing, R. D. *The Politics of Experience.* Ballantine, New York, p. 136, 1967.

Ludwig, A., Levine, J., and Stark, L. H. *LSD and Alcoholism.* Charles Thomas, Springfield, Ill., (1970).

McDonald, N. "Living with Schizophrenia." *Canad. Med. Assoc. J.,* Vol. 82, pp. 218–221, 1960.

Osmond, H., and Smythies, J. R. "Schizophrenia: A New Approach." *J. Ment. Sci.,* Vol. 98, pp. 309–315, 1952.

Taylor, B. "Visions of Hashish." In *The Drug Experience,* D. Ebin, Editor. Grove Press, New York, p. 41 (1965).

Chapter 4

Bleuler, E. *Dementia Praecox or the Group of Schizophrenias.* International U. Press, New York, 1950.

Heston, L. L. "Psychiatric Disorders in Foster-Home-Reared Children of Schizophrenic Mothers." *British Journal of Psychiatry,* Vol. 112, pp. 819–825, 1966.

Kallman, J. *The Genetics of Schizophrenia.* Augustin, New York, 1938.

Kety, S. S., Rosenthal, D., Wender, P. H., and Schulsinger, K. F. "The Types and Prevalence of Mental Illness in the Biological and Adoptive Families of Adopted Schizophrenics." In *The Transmission of Schizophrenia,* D. Rosenthal and S. S. Kety, editors, Pergamon Press, New York, 1968, pp. 345–362.

Pollin, W., and Stabenau, J. R. "Biological, Psychological and

Historical Differences in a Series of Monozygotic Twins Discordant for Schizophrenia." In *The Transmission of Schizophrenia*, D. Rosenthal and S. S. Kety, editors, Pergamon Press, New York, 1968, pp. 317–332.

Chapter 5
Benjamin, J. D. "A Method for Distinguishing and Evaluating Formal Thinking Disorders in Schizophrenia." In *Language and Thought in Schizophrenia*, J. S. Kasanin, editor, Norton, New York, 1964, pp. 65–90.

Bleuler, E. *Dementia Praecox or the Group of Schizophrenias.* International U. Press, New York, 1950, pp. 9; 40; 41.

Goldstein, K., and Scheerer, M. "Abstract and Concrete Behavior." *Psychological Monographs*, Vol. 53, No. 239, 1941.

Chapter 6
Bleuler, E. *Dementia Praecox or the Group of Schizophrenias.* International U. Press, New York, 1950, pp. 54; 55; 56; 97.

Laing, R. D. *Knots.* Pantheon, New York, 1970, pp. 2; 12.

Slater, E., and Roth, M. *Clinical Psychiatry.* Williams & Wilkins, Baltimore, 1969, pp. 273.

Chapter 7
Hoch, P. H., and Polatin, P. "Pseudoneurotic Forms of a Schizophrenia." *Psychiatric Quarterly*, Vol. 23, pp. 248–296, 1949.

Chapter 8
Chapman, J. "The Early Symptoms of Schizophrenia." *British Journal of Psychiatry*, Vol. 112, pp. 225–251, 1966.

Elkes, J. "Schizophrenic Disorder in Relation to Levels of Neuralorganization: The Need for Some Conceptual Points of Reference." In *The Chemical Pathology of the Nervous System*, J. Folch-Pi, editor, Pergamon Press, London, 1961, pp. 648–665.

Hernandez-Peon, R., Sherrer, H., and Jouvet, M. "Modification of Electrical Activity in Cochlear Nucleus During 'Attention' in Unanesthetized Cats." *Science*, Vol. 123, pp. 331–332, 1956.

Lang, P. J., and Buss, A. H. "Psychological Deficit in Schizophrenia. II. Interference and Activation." *Journal of Abnormal Psychology*, Vol. 70, pp. 77–106, 1965.

McDonald, N. "The Other Side: Living with Schizophrenia." *Canadian Medical Association Journal*, Vol. 82, pp. 218–221, 1960.

Mednick, S. A., and Schulsinger, F. "Some Premorbid Characteristics Related to Breakdown in Children with Schizophrenic Mothers." D. Rosenthal and S. S. Kety, editors, Pergamon Press, London, 1968, pp. 267–291.

Ornitz, E. M. "Disorders of Perception Common to Early Infantile Autism and Schizophrenia." In *The Schizophrenic Syndrome*, Vol. 1, pp. 652–671, Brunner/Mazel, Inc., New York, 1971.

Shakow, D. "Segmental Set: A Theory of the Formal Psychological Deficit in Schizophrenia." *Archives of General Psychiatry*, Vol. 6, pp. 1–17, 1961.

Chapter 9

"Benzedrine Alert," *Air Surgeons Bulletin*, Vol. 1, pp. 19–21, 1944, cited in Ray, O. S., *Drugs, Society and Human Behavior* (Mosby, St. Louis, Missouri, 1972, p. 196).

Ellinwood, E. H. "Assault and Homicide Association with Amphetamine Abuse." *American Journal of Psychiatry*, Vol. 127, pp. 1170–1175, 1971.

Freud, S. "On the General Effects of Cocaine." *Medicinisch-chirurgisches Central-Blatt*, Vol. 20, pp. 374–375, August, 1885, reprinted in *Drug Dependence*, Vol. 5, p. 15, 1970.

———, (July 1884:) "On Coca." *Heitler's Centralblatt für die Gesamte Theraphie*, quoted in Jones, E., *ibid.*, p. 82.

Grinspoon, L. "Amphetamines Reconsidered." *Saturday Review*, July 8, 1972.

Jones, E. *The Life and Work of Sigmund Freud* (Basic Books, New York), pp. 80; 84; 82; 81 (1953).

Kramer, J. C., Fischman, V. S., and Littlefield, D. C. "Amphetamine Abuse: Pattern and Effects of High Doses Taken Intravenously." *Journal of the American Medical Association*, Vol. 201, pp. 89–93, 1967.

Lewin, L. *Phantastica: Narcotic and Stimulating Drugs*. Trubner Ltd., London, pp. 80; 76 (1931).

Masaki, T. "The Amphetamine Problem in Japan." *World Health Organization Technical Reports Service*, Vol. 102, pp. 14–19, 1956, cited in Angrist, B. M., and Gershon, S. "Amphetamine Abuse in New York City, 1966–1968." *Seminars in Psychiatry*, Vol. 1, pp. 195–207, 1969.

Monroe, R. R., and Drell, H. J. "All Use of Stimulants Obtained from Inhalers." *Journal of the American Medical Association*, Vol. 135, p. 908, 1947.

Sheehy, G. *Speed Is of the Essence.* Pocketbooks, New York, p. 22 (1971).

Chapter 10
Angrist, B. M., and Gershon, S. "The Phenomenology of Experimentally Induced Amphetamine Psychosis: Preliminary Observations." *Biological Psychiatry*, Vol. 2, pp. 97–107 (1970).

Burroughs, W., Jr. *Speed* (Olympia Press, New York), 1970, pp. 144 and 168.

Connell, T. H. *Amphetamine Psychosis.* Oxford University Press, London, p. 46 (1958).

————. "Amphetamine Psychosis, a Description of the Individuals and Process." *Journal of Nervous and Mental Diseases*, Vol. 144, pp. 273–283, 1967.

Griffith, J. D., Cavanaugh, J., Held, N. N., Oates, J. A. "Dextroamphetamine: Evaluation of Psychotomimetic Properties in Man." *Archives of General Psychiatry*, Vol. 26, pp. 97–100, 1972.

Janowsky, D. S., El-yousef, M. K., Davis, J. M., and Serkerke, H. J. "Provocation of Schizophrenic Symptoms by Intravenous Methylphenidate." *Archives of General Psychiatry*, Vol. 28, p. 185, 1973.

Chapter 12
Aghajanian, G. K., Bunney, S. S., and Kuhar, M. J. "Use of Single Unit Recording in Correlating Transmitter Turnover with Impulse Flow in Monoamine Neurons." In *New Concepts in Neurotransmitter Regulation,* A. J. Mandell, editor, New York, Plenum Press, in press.

Angrist, B. M., Shopsin, B., and Gershon, S. "The Comparative Psychotomimetic Effects of Stereoisomers of Amphetamine." *Nature*, Vol. 234, pp. 152–154, 1971.

Arnold, L. E., Wender, P. H., McCloskey, K., and Snyder, S. H. "Levoamphetamine and Dextroamphetamine: Comparative Efficacy in the Hyperkinetic Syndrome; Assessment by Target Symptoms." *Archives of General Psychiatry*, Vol. 27, pp. 816–822, 1972.

Axelrod, J. "The Metabolism Storage and Release of Catecholamines." *Recent Progress in Hormone Research,* Vol. 21, pp. 597–622, 1965.

Carlsson, A., and Lindqvist, M. "Effect of Chlorpromazine or Haloperidol on the Formation of 3-Methoxyramine and Normetanephrine in Mouse Brain." *Acta Pharmacologica et Toxicologica,* Vol. 20, pp. 140–144, 1963.

Creese, I., and Iversen, S. D. "Amphetamine Response in Rat after Dopamine Neuron Destruction." *Nature,* Vol. 238, pp. 247–248, 1972.

Guth, P. S., and Spirtes, M. A. "The Phenothiazine Tranquilizers: Biochemical and Biophysical Actions." *International Review of Neurobiology,* Vol. 7, pp. 231–278, 1963.

Nyback, H., Borzecki, Z., and Sedvall, G. "Accumulation and Disappearance of Catecholamines Formed from Tyrosine-C in Mouse Brain; Effect of Some Psychotropic Drugs." *European Journal of Pharmacology,* Vol. 4, pp. 395–402, 1968.

Snyder, S. H. "Catecholamines in the Brain as Mediators of Amphetamine Psychosis." *Archives of General Psychiatry,* Vol. 27, pp. 169–179, 1972.

———. "New Developments in Brain Chemistry: Catecholamine Metabolism and Its Relationship to the Mechanism of Action of Psycholotropic Drugs." *American Journal of Orthopsychiatry,* Vol. 37, pp. 864–879, 1967.

———, and Meyerhoff, J. L., "How Amphetamine Acts in Minimal Brain Dysfunction." *Annals of the New York Academy of Sciences,* Vol. 205, pp. 310–320, 1973.

Stein, L. "Self-Stimulation of the Brain and the Central Stimulant Actions of Amphetamine." *Federation Proceedings,* Vol. 23, pp. 836–850, 1964.

Ungerstedt, U. "Stereotaxic Mapping of the Monoamine Pathways in the Rat Brain." *Acta Physiologica Scandinavica,* Vol. 367, Supplement 10, pp. 1–48, 1971.

Appendix 2

Cole, J. O. and Davis, J. M. "Antipsychotic Drugs." In *The Schizophrenic Syndrome,* H. Solomon, editor, New York, Grune and Stratton, pp. 478–568, 1969.

Horn, A. S., and Snyder, S. H. "Chlorpromazine and Dopamine: Conformational Similarities That Correlate with the Antischizophrenic Activity of Phenothiazine Drugs." *Proceedings of the National Academy of Sciences,* U.S.A., Vol. 68, pp. 2325–2328, 1971.

Index

Catalog

If you are interested in a list of fine Paperback
books, covering a wide range of subjects
and interests, send your name and address,
requesting your free catalog, to:

McGraw-Hill Paperbacks
1221 Avenue of Americas
New York, N.Y. 10020